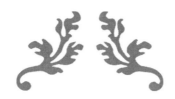

PASSION TO PURPOSE

The Self-Care Anthology

COPYRIGHT 2018
NURSING ON PURPOSE
MARSHANELL MANNING-WRIGHT AND CO-AUTHORS

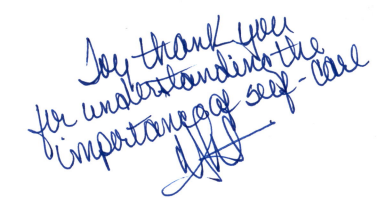

Joy thank you for understanding the importance of self-care

Dedication

This book is dedicated to all the leaders that believed in my potential and saw in me what I did not see in myself. To every person – know that you must believe in yourself first and others will follow and love you enough to put yourself first. To my parents, Henry and Barbara Manning, thank you for your continued support in everything I do.

Acknowledgement

Thank you to my family, especially my grand daughter, for supporting me through this project with your summer visit. We were able to hang out and do a little during this project.

Thank you to every author who has contributed to this anthology - your testimonies will encourage and inspire others to greatness. Thank you to Michelle for supporting and mentoring me through this project.

Love, Marshanell

Table of Contents

Chapter 1 1
   Purpose Driven 2
   Self care in health care 6

Chapter 2 11
   Delayed yet right on time 12
   Self Care 18

Chapter 3 23
   Sorry, Not Sorry 24
   The Race is Not Given to the Swift 33

Chapter 4 43
   From the South Side to the Bed Side 44
   In the Beginning 45
   Growth and Development 50
   Daily Affirmation 52
   Courage and Strength 53
   Self-Reflection 56
   Self-Discovery 58
   Self-Care 60
   End of the Road 63

Chapter 5 67
   When I Found My Voice 68
   Self-Love, Self-Discipline, Self-Respect 73

Chapter 6 79

    The Calling 80

    Nursing as a Spiritual Practice 88

Chapter 7 99

    From CNA to Entrepreneur 100

    Self-care & Self-Love 109

Chapter 8 115

    Lil' Lisa 116

Chapter 9 121

    Poised on Purpose 122

    My Perfect Peace 129

Chapter 10 135

    Let's Talk Rules 136

    I'm Gonna Let It Shine 148

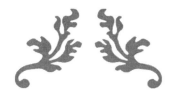

CHAPTER 1

Purpose Driven

As a little girl, I would play often by myself, speaking to my dog "Duke" who was a German shepherd, while the other neighborhood children played outside around the corner. They would play kickball, red light green light, hopscotch or just hang out. Often they would come to our house and want popsicles and to play on our swing set in the back yard. It seems like I have always been different, or I would say focused - not perfect - but focused. My dad and one of his friends had their own security guard business and this is where I got my entrepreneurial spirit.

I remember one time my favorite aunt, Maxine, said I talked a lot; can you believe that, lol? She said that one time I talked so much that she told me to go into my grandmother's walk in closet and then closed the door. She thought this would cause me to be quiet and maybe fall asleep, but when she went back to get me, several hours later, guess what? I was still talking! Remember purpose!

I grew up in Gary, Indiana, which was thriving - we had the United States Steel Mill and people were always coming and going. We loved Saturday mornings; we would go downtown with my grandmother and my Aunt Maxine and eat and shop. It was so much fun and I looked forward to seeing my cousins on both my mother's and my father's side. I would tend to hang around my grandmother while my cousins played. Not understanding my journey and why I would make some of the decisions I would make in the future. When I was in the 10th grade, I got very sick. I had rheumatic fever, which could be very serious and cause

Chapter 1

permanent damage to the heart, including damaged heart valves and heart failure. Rheumatic fever is an inflammatory disease that can develop as a complication of inadequately treated strep throat or scarlet fever. Strep throat and scarlet fever are caused by an infection with streptococcus bacteria (Mayo Clinic, 2017). I was hospitalized for a week and missed about 2 weeks of school. For an adolescent, this was horrible. I wanted to get back to school quickly, but I was still healing. My doctor said that I would have to take antibiotics for the rest of my life…hmm…that was not something I wanted to do! I also remember him wanting to put me on anxiety medication…that did not happen. While in high school, my mother made sure I was focused I always knew as a little girl that I wanted to be a nurse and a teacher, always. So, focused I was, I would meet with my school counselor and take classes that would help me get into nursing school. While some of my friends took the easy classes, I was taking chemistry, biology and other classes to help prepare me for college.

I was ready for college, and to start nursing school…and guess what? Newfound freedom away from home and I get pregnant. I always knew I would be a nurse and a teacher. My road had shifted and now my journey would take a little longer, but when you have a purpose, nothing can stop you but you, and that was not about to happen. I was so scared to tell my parents that I was pregnant; I knew they would be disappointed in me. But I also knew that I would continue to pursue my dream and become a nurse and a teacher. My father said I would never go back to school, yet I knew I would. It was very important to me to show my mother and father (and myself) that I would finish. Remember: purpose!

When I left home and moved to Mountain View, California, I got a job working at Taco Bell making $3.50/hour. I was so happy to get that job; I was only 21 and had no experience whatsoever. I was offered the position of Assistant Manager at Taco Bell and I took it. But soon after this, when I was offered the Manager position, I quickly said no! While attending school to get my Associate Degree in Nursing (ADN), I got my Certified Nursing Assistant (CNA) certificate, left Taco Bell and moved toward my vision of working at a local hospital. After about 15 years, I decided to go back to school to obtain my BSN. During this time, I was pregnant with my 2nd child and the doctors at Stanford Hospital wanted to do an echocardiogram on my heart - because of having rheumatic fever when I was younger, they wanted to make sure I was okay. Well…the echocardiogram was done and if I had not told them I had rheumatic fever, they would not have known there were no signs! Heart valves were great! I stopped taking the antibiotics because I knew I did not need them (I was told by my primary physician I would have to take antibiotics for the rest of my life); remember: purpose! Pregnant with my 3rd child, I continued on for my Masters in Management and Leadership (MSN) and now Doctorate of Nursing Practice (DNP). I was the only one stopping me; I was focused and was not stopping. #Dontstop

Later on in life, I began to see that because I was put in the closet to be quiet, as I got older, I would see something, know something and would not speak up. I began to understand that

Chapter 1

what happens in our childhood affects us in adulthood. Once I saw that this affected me, I could confront it and now take up my authority. I know that I am called to speak and help others, and inspire them to greatness.

As I reflect back on where I came from and where I am now, I see more clearly and understand even more that I have always been purpose driven. Drive is in me, and so engrained it is something I cannot articulate. I give and give and it was hard for me to say no to others because I love to give and care for others - so much so, that I was not doing such a great job for myself. I got over being worried if someone would say I was being selfish because I knew, deep in my heart, I was not. I cannot give what I don't have. I had to learn not only for my personal life, but my work life, as well, and that balance is important. I had to learn to not feel guilty. Turning my cell phone off or on mute, not getting on my computer and stealing away became my friend. Stepping away, getting in a quiet space, listening to the waves and smelling the ocean is very enjoyable for me, as I am able to refresh, regroup and reflect during this sacred time.

Life happens and my father was diagnosed with Dementia in 2016 and passed away May 10, 2018. I knew more than ever that I needed to have time where I could steal away, reflect and care for myself. This weighed heavily on my mother and I knew, as a health care professional/daughter, I had to help my mother get through this time. This is when I got the vision to do "Nursing with Purpose."

Self care in health care

We live in a fast paced world and everything being instant, more demands, working the lean way, more with less. Being a health care professional now for over 20 years, I have seen nurses stressed more, overwhelmed and being verbally abused by patients. Being proactive and caring for one's self is important in order to care for our patients and others. Nurses are now mentally exhausted from the changes that are in healthcare and the stressors that are involved. Nurses are now also experiencing increased stress because of increased work hours and patient workloads.

The term "self care" simply means caring for oneself by exercising, taking a mental health day if needed, doing things that make you happy and sometimes turning off your cell phone. Nurses are drawn into the profession because they feel they have been called and have a strong sense of compassion and empathy. Because of a nurse's dedication to help others at their most vulnerable time, we tend to neglect our own health and self care needs. All health care workers are at risk for having burnout and we must seek out ways to avoid burnout. Self care is becoming more and more an awareness to health care professionals to prevent burnout. Addressing the total person - physically, emotionally, mentally and spiritually is important. While working, we are expected not to bring the emotional and spiritual part to our workplace. Emotional and spiritual health are both relevant to mental and physical aspects of life; an example would be that exercising helps release serotonin, which is a hormone in the brain that helps provide a feeling of well being. I propose to care for myself first, so that I can effectively care for others; I have a servant's heart no matter where I am.

I cherish my early mornings when it is quiet and I can hear the birds chirping and wind blowing. This is the time where I get ideas and can hear from God. For me, it is important to steal away and have the quiet that I need to recharge, refresh and regroup. Being a giver at heart, and wanting to help others, I have to make sure that I give back to myself, taking charge of my life and not saying yes because I feel obligated or guilty. I have watched some of my family and friends quality of life worsen due to lack of self-care and understanding that the body can only do so much, I feel my responsibility is to help them.

As a professional healthcare worker, addressing the total person is important. I aim to care for myself by exercising, deciding what I will allow in my space and keeping myself around other inspiring people with positive vibes. As a little girl, I would often play by myself and just did not surround myself around a lot of people. As I have gotten older and more mature, I now realize that quiet time and stealing away to refresh, regroup and recharge in my profession is important. I believe that God was preparing me, even as a child, because He is all knowing. I learned to love myself and be okay with myself and who I am created to be. Once this happened I began to see things happening in my life.

Family is important to me, I learned this from my grandmother and mom, I love to cook and turn it into a party because everyone takes their minds off of what is going on at that time and enjoy themselves, this is apart of caring for yourself and others. I love hanging out with my friends, whether it be on the phone or in person, we can always offer encouragement and have our girlfriend/sister time.

Taking care of yourself first, whether it is attending to your personal upkeep, exercising, being still and having a massage, allows for you to be healed. Addressing mind, body, soul and the total person, is key and it starts with me.

#SELF-CAREINHEALTHCARE

#IAMTHECHANGE.

Chapter 1

About the Author

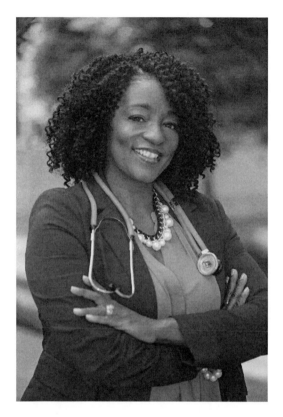

Marshanell Wright, DNP, MSN, BSN, PHN is a trailblazer in her profession. Originally from Gary, Indiana, she now resides in San Jose, California. Marshanell works collaboratively with other leaders in her discipline. A forward thinker and strategist, she leads by empowering others to make decisions while motivating through consensus building. Furthermore, she engages her staff by explaining the "why" and leads by example.

In 2011, Marshanell received the Award of Excellence. She was then awarded with the Leadership Development Diversity Program recognition in 2013. She has been recognized as a committed leader that focuses on being an agent of change within the health care industry. Marshanell is intrigued with the challenges of combining technology & nursing. Her ultimate goal is to make technology more end-user friendly and simplistic so that nurses can focus more on patients and less on a technological device. Moreover, her aspirations are to continue mentoring, inspiring, teaching and encouraging others to excel in their career/life. Marshanell has given a focus on "What about the Nurse," a topic of concern addressing the concerns and needs of nurses from their day-to-day care of their patients.

During her downtime, Marshanell enjoys reading, going to the ocean, jogging, traveling and listening to music, educating and empowering nurses and women. This has led Marshanell into starting her own business - Nursing on Purpose LLC and Women Empowering Women.

Contact Information:

Email: purposedrivennurse@gmail.com
IG: https://www.instagram.com/purposedrivennurse
Cell: 408-490-3433

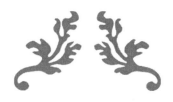

CHAPTER 2

Delayed yet right on time

I know it may seem cliché to say; however, since I was a little girl, I wanted to be a nurse. I kept those play toy doctor and nurse kits and would faithfully practice "listening" to their hearts and giving them shots. I remember explaining to my dolls that I had to give them a shot. I would tell my dolls to be brave, that it would hurt just for a second.

My childhood was very challenging; more often than not, I found myself attempting to console myself the same way as I would pretend to with my dolls. As time passed, life and responsibilities seemed to put a damper on my childhood dream of becoming a nurse. My first job, at the age of 14, at the local grocery store, wasn't what I expected. In high school, my sister and I literally ran a local seafood restaurant, called Captain D's, after school until closing. Football season, my sister and I were on the cheerleading team. In my junior and senior years of high school, I worked at a nursing home as a nurse aid. I was so excited to be working as an aid, as I felt this was the first part of the process of me getting into nursing school.

I graduated from high school and it was time for college. At this point in my life, I had only had one boyfriend, and shortly after my freshman year in college, I met what ended up being my husband. My major at the time was in healthcare, but it was not nursing as I wanted it to be. I put college on hold as I had ended up getting married very young, moving to Florida and had my first child within the first year. My pregnancy was considered "high risk" and I was unable to work, so I picked back up some college courses and became a "homemaker." I was so excited to get back to work after having my son and even more excited to finally use my degree in healthcare, which I was able to complete during my pregnancy, because I switched my major to being a registered medical assistant. This made me happy but only for a while, because I was restricted on what I could do and what I could not do. In my heart, I was sad because I wanted desperately to be a nurse; it just didn't seem it was possible for me because I had to work to help pay bills, be a wife and a mother. It never seemed like there was ever a "right time" for me to go back to school to fulfill my dream of becoming a nurse. The years passed, and I had another child and then LIFE HAPPENED. The very thing that was my worst nightmare became my reality…my husband left our small children and me and then asked for a divorce.

I should have seen this coming and I'm certain my spirit had prepared for it because I wasn't shocked when it happened, more so caught off guard at the timing. Literally, my life propelled deeper into a mixture of feelings of failure, numbness and sheer determination to NEVER put myself in the position to depend on anyone when it came to the security of my finances and a roof over my and my children's head. I knew he wasn't coming back, so after about six months of trying to stabilize myself and my children, I left the state and caught a plane back home to Ohio with the clothes on my back and one suitcase for each of my children. I felt like such a burden, having to move back home with my parents with my small children. The adjustment was rocky in many ways. I signed up for nursing school and got started working within the first two months of relocating back to Ohio. I asked myself repeatedly what in the world I was thinking and now was definitely not the time to go back to school because I had bills to pay. I felt the doubt and the "side eye" looks from people around me, but I didn't care - I was determined to get my RN degree no matter what.

About four to five months after living in Ohio and having a job, I was able to move out of my parents' house into a very small apartment for my children and I. Shortly thereafter, I was in my first semester of nursing school. A year later, my sister and I were in the courtroom and the judge called my name. I went up to the judge's panel with my sister by my side as he lowered his voice some and gave the official speech and all I remembered hearing him say was, "I hereby grant you the divorce from xxxx on this day and this year," and he slammed the gavel down and I felt numb as my sister hugged me and silent tears fell from both of our cheeks. That was the first time I allowed myself to shed a tear and yet felt almost nothing. I had work to do.

Fast forward two more years, my last semester of nursing school. I was exhausted. I was working at the hospital from 7:00 am to 7:00 pm, and the days I wasn't working, I had class or clinical. For three years, I had maybe one day off here and there. My life consisted of my children's schoolwork, my job and nursing school. That was our life, day in and day out. My sister always helped me when she could and would even take time off from her job whenever one of my boys got sick. My youngest two children have severe asthma, so I was always walking on thin ice with my attendance for work and school. I knew something had to give, so I made the dreaded decision of moving back in with my parents for my last semester of nursing, because I just could not keep up working full time or part time and be able to finish nursing school, because at this point in the last semester, I had clinical and/or class every day. I was going to drop the ball. I was unraveling mentally, physically and emotionally and something had to give. I got on the phone and called the kids' grandparents in Florida and told them I needed their help with the boys. The next week they were there to pick them up. To this day, that was the hardest decision I've ever made - to look into my oldest son's eyes as he wailed, begging me not to make him. He was also worried about who would take care of me, with him being gone. I reassured him the best I could that it was only a few months and I'd send for them.

Four months later, I was taking the exit exam to get out of nursing school and I failed it by three points. I was devastated, to say the least, yet determined to graduate on time. I had a chance to take the exit exam one more time before the semester ended. I took the test, clicked on "submit" and it immediately showed that I passed with a 97%. I was elated but I knew I wasn't finished - it was time to prepare for the state boards. I took a date about a month after my graduation pinning ceremony, which was bittersweet because I had always imagined my oldest son being the one to pin me; but he wasn't able to be there due to my circumstances. I had my sister there and she was the next best honor that I had to pin me.

The day before my boards, I had just gotten back in town from visiting my boys and just wanted to get it over with. I looked at a few notes and left it at that. The morning of the exam I was seated at the computer at 8:40 am. The board's test question had me at bit baffled at the way the questions were asked, so I literally read each question and answer once and chose the first answer that came to mind. I noticed I was in the question number 70 so I continued to answer a few more questions and after question 75 my computer screen literally went blank. I sat there stunned and almost panicked thinking to myself either I nailed it in a good way or the computer thought I was a dummy and had enough of my wrong answers. I glanced at the clock when I got in my car and saw it was only 9:20 am. I threw my head into my hands and just knew I failed because I was barely there an hour.

The next two days was a blur. I spent those days at my sister's house. I was a wreck. I was mentally sick with worry as I waited for the test results. I tried to keep myself busy because I had just gotten the boys and me a new place, so I was getting it ready for their return in a few weeks. Yes, I did all the tricks and even paid money to get results early, only to get the results within a few hours of each other. I was sitting on my sister's bed, talking to her on day two, post taking the test. I casually checked my email and there it was. I had an email from the Ohio Board of Nursing congratulating me for passing the boards and giving me my license number. I looked at my sister and said "OMG, I PASSED!" My sister hugged me, and as I walked to the bathroom, it felt as if a dam broke and I literally fell to my knees thanking GOD as the tears came and flooded uncontrollably. It was the first time in almost four years that I cried and felt EVERYTHING.

Chapter 2

In that moment, everything I had gone through to get to that point burst through my heart and soul. It came pouring out. All those days and nights I would have to drop my kids off to daycare at 5:00 am and not pick them up till 8:00 pm, because I had to work or go to school, crushed my heart because I felt like I was hurting them by not getting to spend quality time with them. I would get home make them food and sometimes not even eat myself because I was too tired; just to turn around and do it all over again the next day. The hurt from the previous marriage, the divorce, and everything I went through in between, came to the surface. I was able to finally begin to DEAL with all that I had experienced up to that point, so that I could finally HEAL.

I made it happen. I prayed often and gave it all I could. You can do ANYTHING you put your mind to if you BELIEVE you can. I did. I know in my heart that with God, and sheer determination on your part, anything is possible - and I'm a living testimony of just that.

Self Care

As we go through the hustle and bustle of everyday life, many of us often neglect the physical, spiritual and emotional needs of the most important person - you! There are endless amounts of responsibilities and things on our "to-do" list, so it feels that the job is never done right. Self-care is something that I've struggled with and had a hard time incorporating into my life. I would find myself very tired on all levels and lacked motivation while I continued to put myself last. I began to realize that I was tapping out at times from an empty place because I wasn't taking the time to care for myself and fill myself back up physically, spiritually and emotionally. I became mindful of this and determined to find a way to give myself the same care and love that I constantly poured into others; this was life changing for me. I started off small by setting aside a time in the evenings for myself to do something - at least one thing I enjoyed, which is reading. Once I was able to be consistent with that, I added some self-care to my weekly routine, which seemed a little more difficult to do, and that is listening to music while stretching. It may seem daunting; however, the rewards of taking time for yourself to settle your mind, rejuvenate your body and doing something to make yourself happy are indeed priceless!

I have listed below some self-care examples that I've used, as well as others I know. I hope this helps someone, and please remember...you're worth it! Self -Care examples:

- Listen to your favorite music
- Take a relaxing bath
- Go for a walk, jog or run
- Get enough sleep that's best for YOUR body
- Watch a movie or go see a comedy
- Ask for help when needed
- Choose attire that makes you feel good
- Pray and/or sit silently and allow your thoughts to slow down
- Be mindful of the foods you eat
- Take a "daycation"
- Be around positive people and those you love and that display the same in return
- Love yourself

About The Author

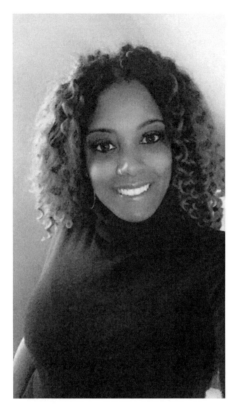

Ashley Ramos, RN, ACRN is a native of Columbus, Ohio and resides there with her children. She has been working in healthcare for over a decade and completed her dream of becoming an RN in 2016. Since then, she has been working as an Acute Care Registered Nurse at a local hospital in Columbus. Although Ashley loves her career as a Registered Nurse, she quickly realized that it was just the foundation laid for her higher purpose in life. She is currently pursing, and is near completion, of her certification as a Holistic Wellness coach while working towards opening her business named "The Solace Place LLC " that is a place that focuses on holistic wellbeing, inner peace, rest, rejuvenation and tranquility.

She has a passion for inner peace, sound mind, education and advocating for patients needs. In her free time she enjoys spending time with her children, spoken word, salsa dancing and reading literature.

To contact the author:

Email: r_ashlie33@yahoo.com

CHAPTER 3

Sorry, Not Sorry

I have always been a people pleaser and wanted to fit in. Ever since I was an elementary school student, I remember wanting to ensure that everyone was content with me. Whether it was family, teachers, church family, parents of friends or even the popular girls at the school, I wanted everyone to like me. Growing up in a small town, where the black population wasn't nearly as recognized as its counterparts, I wanted to prove that not only could I be just as great, but also likeable. I was an observant student in that I studied the actions of people that were the most admired. I would try to imitate their movements and my attempts failed miserably. On top of growing up in a small town, I attended a Catholic school for most of my elementary years. At one point, I was the only black kid in the entire school. As anyone can imagine, there was a ton of pressure on me to be the perfect model. Not only did I have to be a super achiever in the academic realm, but I also had to exude my idea of all the traits of the perfect young lady. I remember already being viewed as different and being told that I couldn't be friends with some of my classmates because I was black. I would get questioned about why my hair felt different and why my skin was darker. My esteem would peak when my hair was straightened. I could twirl my hair around and "blend" in like the other girls at school and I knew they were elated to see me with a comparable style. We would play outside at recess and I would love the feeling of my hair bouncing up and down and I would catch myself imitating my friends. However, as soon as I walked past the mirror in the bathroom, I was reminded that I was still a black girl, as curls

Chapter 3

would start to form. My straight hair might have lasted two days and then I was back to braids and being questioned why my hair was once again different.

My most vivid memory circles around picture day in second grade. My mom had combed my hair in a different style and I knew better than to even touch it until the photos were over. On picture day, the photographer provided cheap black combs for everyone prior to getting their photos taken. I would look around and notice everyone combing his or her hair and laughing. I didn't touch my hair until right after my photo was complete. I took that cheap comb and pulled it through my curly bangs and that thing got stuck. Not only was I unable to remove the stupid thing, but it was also hanging in front of my face. I had to go the nurse's office because my teacher was scared to touch my greasy hair. The nurse ended up cutting the comb out of my hair. All of this drama over my need to fit in.

I remember wanting to fit in so badly that I asked my mom to convert to Catholicism. Please don't get me wrong; there is absolutely nothing wrong with being Catholic, but it was a shocking moment to my mother because I was raised African Methodist Episcopal. I liked my church and the people in it, but in order to be like my classmates, I wanted to convert and attend church with them. Not only was I the only black kid in the school, but I was also one of the few who were not Catholic. That meant on Mondays and Wednesdays when we attended mass, I wasn't allowed to take communion. The priests made it so obvious and I once again was questioned why I was different.

Throughout middle school, high school and college, I continually strived to fit in and please everyone around me. I would dress the way I thought I was expected, talk in the manner that was socially acceptable and even act in a way that would be presentable to the masses. In my mind, I was put together, but in reality I was a hot mess. It was so bad that a couple of teachers had pulled me to the side to make sure I was okay. I guess the internal struggle was real.

Going into the workforce, I learned to play the game. My immediate strategy was to go into the office and fit in. I would learn which managers needed to be impressed the most and my mission to please was in full motion. I would learn the culture and adapt myself into being what I thought the company would want me to be. Little did I realize that this game I was putting myself in was a career jail. I was keeping everyone happy, and smiled through the fakeness, every single day. As soon as I walked to my car and got in, my smile would erase and I would go through how unhappy I was. I truly thought my "Operation Make Everyone Happy with You" game was the way to succeed. Unfortunately, I was remaining stagnant in my career.

Being a mother only added to this falsehood of reality that I thought was expected. Understand that, in my mind, adding a kid to the equation meant that I not only had to prove to my peers that I could appear as supporting partner, career woman and a mommy, but that I could also hold it all together. On top of that, I had to show my family that I knew how to be a successful mother. The worst of all was trying to keep appearances with the elite parents of my daughter's daycare. It was by God's grace that

Chapter 3

we were able to afford our daughter's expensive school, but in my mind I had to prove that we were able to fit in and were just as special. In the afternoons, I would ride the elevator up to her school and stand up extra straight and check my phone. In my mind, I was proving to the other parents that I was just as important and successful as they were. I promise I am not crazy, but this is really how I operated each day. Exhausting, right?

Well, my approach to the way that I lived life changed dramatically on New Year's Day, 2018. I was on the plane with my husband and daughter on our way back from our holiday break in California. As you can probably tell, my mind constantly races and it feels like it never turns off. Being on a plane for over five hours where I am limited to thinking and sitting still allows me to plan, my daughter and her children's futures. Not really, but kind of. My husband always tells me to "rest my brain," but I feel that challenge is nearly impossible. It was on this flight I remember having the epiphany that led me to where I am today.

I typically create a New Year's resolution every year, to please anyone who asks. I feel that resolutions are something forced because society has always pressured that belief. In the past, it would be something like losing weight, saving money or reading a self-help book once a month. I then decided to make my resolution (responses to people) more deep and conversational. Again, still in a response to please others around me. I would state that my resolution was to be happy or strive for excellence in all facets of my life. What did that really mean? I have no idea. So, while on the plane, I realized that the idea of a resolution was not for me. In fact, I also had Oprah's "aha" moment. I had been living my entire life pleasing everyone else and not even stepping back and thinking about what Azzleeta wanted and needed. Where was my self-care?

On this day, I made a promise to myself that I would focus on myself unapologetically. I made this vow and promised that it would focus on all aspects of my life: family, work and friends. The realization that over thirty years of my life had been dedicated to pleasing others, who could really care two craps about me, was almost sickening. I was not living my best life, but was allowing my mind to tell me what others expected in order to fit in and be pleasing on the outside. However, I realized that in the land of smoke and mirrors, the outside appearances were not nearly as important as what I held internally. I know I am a good, spiritually grounded person, but I was not allowing me to be myself.

My epiphany sounded great and it felt right. I just was uncertain of how I was going to execute being unapologetic without being offensive. In this realization, I understood that I was going to have to say no at times. I would also have to speak my mind fearlessly and not be scared of how others would take my response. Most importantly, I had to also understand that not everyone was going to like me and I had to learn that I would survive.

My first step in implementing my newly trained thought process was really deepening my relationship with God. I have always been a believer and prayed, but I was not leaning on Him and turning to Him for guidance. In the past, I would wake up in the morning and thank God for waking me, pray before meals and say a short prayer at night. Of all the blessings I had been provided thus far, I was giving Him the bare minimum in forms of communication.

Chapter 3

What I realized was all of my energy was devoted to those I was trying to please and not the one person who has brought me favor and covered me since birth. I now am a regular communicator with Him. I find myself having regular conversations with Him daily. I constantly tell Him thank you for just being present. God is really the big homie. Now, don't get me wrong, I am still learning each day on how to be a better faithful servant, but I am enjoying my truth and utilizing what God has taught me. It is so important to implement self-care in my life in order to be the truest version of myself.

Growing up in a single parent household, I watched my mom put her needs after her three children and she did a great job raising us. I give her a standing ovation for all of the work that she had put forth in order to successfully raise us. Her life was phased into three parts: children, work and church. I never saw her really enjoy things for herself. I saw myself heading in that same direction. I allowed my husband to put his schedule first and added my daughter's schedule in the mix. Whatever time was left over I would allow for myself. As a mom though, let's be real. After the dinner is completed, homework is finished, bath time is checked off and the kid is in bed, there is no time for anything except prepping for the next day. Wifehood and motherhood are no joke.

I had to have a conversation with my husband and tell him unapologetically that I was tired and did not feel my happiest. From outside appearances, I looked and seemed great, but behind closed doors, I felt like I was evaporating in a black hole. I also told him that I fully intended on changing my thought process by focusing more on myself. Of course, I was fearful in telling him my truth, but following my conversations with God, I knew no matter the outcome, I would be at peace. Surprisingly, my husband shrugged his shoulder and agreed. In fact, he stated that he wanted to see me happier and enjoy life more. He was tired of seeing me try to please others and not live for myself. Apparently, he had been telling me this for years, but I wasn't listening. I do not really recall these conversations, but that is beside the point. With this conversation, my husband and I agreed that I needed to go to the gym often in order to alleviate some of the stress from my crazy workdays. He allowed me to schedule my gym time first and worked around my schedule to accommodate his.

Additionally, after my unapologetic conversation, he became extremely hands on with raising our daughter. Please understand - he is a fantastic father, but I am admittedly a helicopter mom and never gave him the opportunity to parent the way he preferred. I was caught up with the idea of ensuring that we appeared as perfect parents, and in order for the perception to visually appear true, I took charge in the parenting domain. No one is perfect right? I digress, but with allowing him to take a bigger hands-on approach, I have been able to enjoy life more. Being able to be Azzleeta outside of being a wife and mother has made me enjoy being a wife and a mother more. There is nothing like having a girl's night, getting more involved in community service, or having pamper time, all while knowing that home is being taken care of. My personal life has changed dramatically by unapologetically allowing me time to truly focus on being myself.

With my career, I knew that walking into the office and telling my boss that I was tired and planning to focus on myself would end with a pink slip and an escort out of the building. So strategy was definitely necessary in order to be unapologetically me. In corporate America, I fully understand the need to follow certain protocol, but there still had to be a way to follow my promise. Instead of playing the character that I assumed would be required in order to move forward, I started being myself. To my surprise, I was becoming more respected. In fact, I was given opportunities that had never been offered before, and I learned that it is okay to respectfully and professionally give my opinion. I find joy in knowing that I am allowed to speak my opinions without the fear of what colleagues would think about me.

My friendships have enhanced to the tenth degree since refusing to impress others. I have been able to spend quality time with friends and support them in their accomplishments. More importantly, I have had an opening to truly be myself and not feel the need to hold back on conversations I had wanted to have without the fear of my reputation being ruined. Through this, my girlfriends and I have become closer and a true support system has been developed. There is nothing like having a friend to talk to when I am upset with the husband and need a second opinion to hear a different point of view. I love being able to go to a friend's house looking a hot mess and discussing how difficult motherhood can be. It is a wonderful feeling to have a true support group who are there through the tears, laughing at the lame jokes and celebrating the wins. My unapologetic self has created a necessary honesty that has allowed my friendships to be stronger than ever.

I am so proud of me for taking this leap of faith in taking care of me. I no longer require someone's approval in order to move forward in my life. In fact, this new lease on life has me laughing at myself for being such a fool for so long and wanting approval from others. I am truly living my best life and am happy. Blessings are continually flowing in and I credit it to my God granting me the opportunity to really focus on myself. My advice for anyone who asks me what to do regarding self-care is to be unapologetically you. Don't waste time being focused on trying to appease what others would view as okay. Find what makes you happy and live your life to the fullest. At the end of the day, not everyone will like you and some will pretend to like you while having ulterior motives. There will be a time when someone will state that they don't agree with decisions you have made. The best response to that person is, "sorry, not sorry!"

The Race is Not Given to the Swift

When reflecting on my journey, my initial thought is that I don't have much of a story to tell. I am a regular person who has lived a regular life. I highly doubt that Lifetime will be calling me for a made for television movie anytime soon. My life seems pretty average. I do not have the story of walking ten miles to get to school, or overcoming extreme/life threatening obstacles, but what I do know is my journey is special. If I were to draw a visual picture, it would have a few drab colors, mixed with bright hues and a few sparkles incorporated throughout. My journey is not perfect, but I am so thankful for it.

I was born in Houston, Texas to high school sweethearts. My parents were both originally from one of my favorite cities, Meridian, Mississippi. After high school, my father relocated to Houston to join the military. My mom decided to quit college a couple of years after and married my father. She became pregnant with yours truly after the wedding. I don't really remember much about Texas, as we left when I was three. I do have vague memories of riding a bus with my mom and going to her job at a paint shop, I believe. I don't really remember my father being at the house much, but apparently he was present at times. My parents decided to divorce when I was around two or three. I later found out it was because my father became addicted to drugs and was constantly in and out of jail. My mother thought it was best to remove us from the situation. I am thankful that she put us first and chose me over her first love. I can only imagine how difficult of a decision this was for her. Thankfully, my mother came from a solid household with two parents who were phenomenal. My grandmother was an educator and my grandfather was a retired military man who worked his butt off to build a stable home for his family. My grandparents are pretty awesome.

About a year later, my mom reconnected with her college sweetheart and they married in my grandparents' home. It was a very small ceremony. I remember being in their bedroom and looking at my mom in her wedding dress. She seemed happy and looked pretty. I also remember my stepfather's family. They weren't overly excited and didn't smile much. They were also quite different than my mom's side of the family. At the young age of three, I remember clear as day not liking the man that my mom was marrying. In fact, I got popped on the hand for not wanting to hold his hand or take a picture with him. You know how they say that children are innocently honest? That was me. I could not stand that man. But nothing makes a little girl happier than seeing her mom smile.

After the wedding, the three of us moved to North Carolina, where my stepfather had a great job at an IT company. Shortly thereafter, my mom went back to college and completed her degree. I may not be a fan of my stepfather, but I am grateful for him financially helping my mom complete this milestone with two children. Oh, I forgot to mention that she became pregnant with my brother before finishing her degree. My mom received her engineering degree and was employed at the same IT company in North Carolina as my stepfather. We lived there for a couple of years until we relocated to Kokomo, Indiana. My mom and stepfather were both offered promising jobs as engineers for a car manufacturer.

Chapter 3

Kokomo brought exciting times for our family. My stepdad unofficially adopted me and I shared the same last name as everyone in the household. He and my mother bought land and built one of the largest homes in the neighborhood and they had my little sister. My mom and stepdad continued to work and both received their MBA's. My stepdad would coach my brother's basketball team and train us in tennis and track. From an outsider's perspective, we were the perfect family. However, little did I know how evil this man was to my mother. His negativity eventually seeped out to the children, as well.

I remember there was a day we were preparing for a road trip to Oklahoma. My mom and stepfather were having an argument about something. By this time, arguments were a normal part of the day. In order to "hide" their disagreement, they went to the bathroom. The yelling was getting louder and louder and ultimately ended in a loud boom. I found out that he pushed my mother forcefully and caused her to fall in the bathtub. On that day, I made a promise to myself to protect my mother and never let a man raise his hand to me. If he did, there was a guarantee that I would not go down without a fight. The inner gangster in me formed.

The incident that caused me to lose all respect for this man was when I was 14 years old. I was preparing to go on my first college tour and my mom had taken me to the store to buy the essentials and get my glasses fixed. When we got back home, my mom parked on the side of the house so my brother could play basketball in the driveway. All of a sudden, my stepdad stormed out of the house and grabbed my brother's Gameboy out of the glove compartment. He was out in the neighborhood screaming and cursing out my mother for confiscating the video game because she wanted to limit his screen time. My mom tried to hurry into the house, but my stepdad stopped her in the garage. He was directly in her face and at that point, a fire inside of me erupted and Gangsta Boo emerged. I felt like I as in a movie. I pushed my mom back and stood in front of her. I would no longer allow him to disrespect my mom. My stepping up to him ignited even more anger and he lost it. This grown man attempted to swing at me and I was having none of it. All of the anger that I withheld from the day that she married that man through all of the disrespect and stress he caused was let out. I kind of blacked out and let him have it, all while holding my mom back. The only thing that was physically hurt in the end was my glasses, which broke in half.

From there, my stepfather started acting more erratically. He would take my brother, sister and me to the store and tell us that my mom was having affairs with everyone under the sun. He would speak nonsensical messes and was disrespectful to his own children. It got so bad that my mom ultimately had to file for divorce. He had her in and out of courts and tried to have joint custody. What we eventually found out was that my stepfather was fully diagnosed with bipolar disorder. To this day, he is under care at a treatment facility, as he is not mentally well. Please believe when I say, mental illness is real.

After the divorce, my mom continued running the household business as usual. One would never know the pure hell we all had experienced because she refused to let us suffer anymore. My

Chapter 3

brother, sister and I remained heavily involved in school and we were scholars. All three of us were highly respected by our teachers and peers. Each of us graduated with honors from high school and were all accepted into multiple colleges. My mom deserves complete kudos for raising three intelligent children through a major storm and not even pausing in the midst of the craziness.

I attended college in Indiana for a year and did horribly. I had no interest in this school, hated being there and was miserable. My uncle and aunt had requested that I move to Oakland, California to assist with their children. I think everyone could tell I was moving in a downward spiral. All of the stress from my stepdad, and the emotions that I had not dealt with, combined with being depressed in college, caused me to end up in a low place. California opened up my eyes to reality and I treasured what my potential was. I went to a community college and did really well. I utilized my hidden leadership skills and became involved in multiple organizations. My uncle and aunt introduced me to a new way of life and provided me with future goals to aspire to in my future. After completing two years in California, I applied to my dream school, the illustrious Spelman College, and was accepted.

I moved to Atlanta, Georgia in August 2006. Spelman was the best decision I ever made. I entered this new world filled with beautiful black women who all were leaders in their own right. It was so intriguing to notice how much diversity there was within the gates of our small school. It also didn't hurt that Morehouse and Clark were right across the parking lot. Spelman and the Atlanta University Center is where I met my lifelong friends. Also while there, I met a nice young man who I found out was from San Jose, California and was born in Indiana. What in the world? I thought he was making fun of me for living in the Bay Area and being raised in Indiana, but he was serious. This dude appeared to be a thug, but opened his mouth and spoke so eloquently. I was intrigued. I started off as his Spanish tutor, but ended up becoming a "friend." He spoke a good game, but after two months of being "friends," I flipped the script on him and demanded that he and I become a couple. In other words, I threatened him and said he either was going to be my boyfriend or walk away from all of this. Romantic…I know. Needless to say, he made the smart decision and we entered the new phase of coupledom.

For the first time in a long time, I was starting to feel well rounded. I had great friends, an amazing boyfriend and was getting my degree from my dream college. Just a few years ago, I was in the garage exchanging blows with my stepdad. My journey had come so far, but I knew I still had a distance to travel.

I graduated from Spelman and my boyfriend graduated from Morehouse. We both entered the workforce with decent jobs and were traveling outside of the country. The economy was plummeting at the time, and we were broke as a joker, making every dollar count in order to create experiences. He was starting to take off with his job in Sales at major pharmaceutical company and a little money was coming in. I just knew he was about to propose. And then…the company laid him off. It took him a freaking year to find a new job. This translates to another year of me not having a ring. Once he got back on his feet, I knew my day

Chapter 3

was coming. In fact, my twenty-sixth birthday was approaching. My boyfriend told me he had a surprise and I was so excited. He was taking me to a fancy restaurant…at California Pizza Kitchen. I still had hopes as he handed me my gift. It was a card with Fantasia concert tickets. Really though? Fantasia is talented and all, but she isn't a ring. I was pissed and had an internal attitude for the rest of the night. Well, you know how people say, "God doesn't like ugly?" Well, instead of a ring that would last a lifetime that night, I got a child.

So there I was: twenty-six, unmarried and pregnant. I thought the world was coming to an end. I worked for a conservative law firm, came from a well-respected southern family and here I was knocked up. I had planned on scheduling an abortion during the MLK Jr. holiday. However, after guidance from our parents and godparent, we decided to keep the baby. We were mentally and financially unprepared, but realized that we had a blessing growing. Nine months later, our little angel entered the world and our lives changed for the better. I thought I had a lot of sass and energy, but I have nothing on this girl. Not only did our princess bring unfound joy into our lives, she motivated me to work harder as a career woman. I give all of my career success to my daughter, as she made me move out of my comfort zone to find a position I was truly qualified for.

Not everything was roses after having my daughter. I did lose a couple of friends who did not agree with me having her out of wedlock. I was even told that if I had a baby, I wouldn't get married or have my dream wedding. After these conversations, I knew it was time to cut ties with people, because I did not want the negative energy surrounding my new family. Additionally, we refused to put our daughter in a crappy daycare center and placed her in one of the best daycares in Atlanta. We struggled financially, but were able to keep her in the school. God was really watching over us.

After eight years – yes, eight long years - my boyfriend proposed to me. Of course I said yes and we planned our dream wedding in Mexico with family and friends. It was everything I wanted and more. However, I knew that the wedding was just the beginning of our new chapter. I would love to say that it has been a fairytale ever since, but let's be real, relationships are hard work. How can you love someone so much, want to strangle them, but then realize that you would be sad if you hurt him? Am I the only one?

Along with the growth of marriage, I have grown as a professional in my career. It is something powerful to think about where I started in my career and where I am now. It is even crazier to me because I know there are more career opportunities and movements for growth. I recently had a full circle moment when I attended a conference in Washington D.C. I was sitting at a table with a former boss who I now communicate with as a peer. It was a moment that made me pause and tell God thank you.

Speaking of how awesome God is, my father and I reunited shortly after I had my daughter. They immediately bonded and she would cry whenever he tried to put her down. He was newly engaged and a deacon of the church. My father apologized for not being there through my childhood years. He even explained to me that he turned to drugs as a mechanism to heal while fighting abroad. His friend/sergeant was blown up right in front of him in Panama. He had no one to talk to and drugs were the only way to numb the pain. This revelation brought closure and forgiveness in my heart. I realized that my father had his own journey that he traveled. For me, that was growth.

Of course there is still so much more to my journey, but these are the highlights thus far in my life. I have experienced some highs and extremely low lows, but I am so thankful. Every step on my journey has helped to define the person that I am today. My life is nowhere near perfect and I am okay with that. The bright colors overcompensate the drab and the hints of sparkle in my picture represent the constant glimmer of hope that I will continue to hold on to. To be honest, I might actually add a little more shine. As each day continues and more doors open, my faith becomes stronger.

About The Author

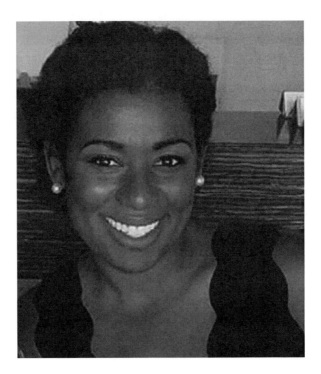

Azzleeta Wright is an HR professional who focuses on immigration and global mobility. She received her B.A. in English from Spelman College. In addition to her career, Azzleeta is an active member of Alpha Kappa Alpha Sorority Incorporated. She is an advocate of enriching the lives of young women and helping them achieve their educational goals. Azzleeta specializes in strategic fundraising, project planning and empowering youth. When not working and volunteering, Azzleeta enjoys traveling and spending time with her husband and daughter.

To Contact the Author:

Email: Azzleetawright@gmail.com

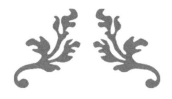

CHAPTER 4

From the South Side to the Bed Side

"Mama, when I grow up, I 'ma be a nurse."

"You gotta study hard and get good grades so you can go to college and be a Registered Nurse; that way, you can give orders instead of take orders."

That conversation happened when I was seven years old, and like every student in my second grade class, I had big dreams of becoming a professional like the people on the posters that hung on the walls of our classroom.

As a child, I spent my summers taking care of the neighborhood kids. I was good at it since I practiced on my four younger siblings. There were eight kids in my family; the first seven all within a nine year period. We were poor and lived in a rundown neighborhood. But life was good because we had a two-parent household and my Dad had a good job working as a janitor for the State of California. That meant we had full medical benefits and visited Kaiser Permanente often enough for me to become intrigued by the nurses who were extremely nice and looked so professional in their starched whites. So, from a very young age, I was influenced to become a Registered Nurse. The road was not always easy, but I never lost sight of the end goal. This is my journey.

In the Beginning

All through elementary, junior high and high school, I got good grades. School was easy for me; I had a great memory and a fairly high IQ. Most of the time, I was bored in class and spent quite a bit of my day irritating the teacher after completing my assignments in record time. My junior year of high school, I met with my counselor to share my plans for college. Since I had a fairly high GPA (3.7) and SAT score, I assumed I would receive the same college advice as my white counterparts regarding college applications and scholarships. Instead, my counselor advised me to become a Certified Nurse Assistant, rather than a Registered Nurse, so I could begin working in as little as 3 months. That way, I could help out my mother financially and not be a burden. I was confused and disappointed and it was very difficult to accept that my counselor was giving me advice not to attend college. This was my first roadblock as an African American female of low socioeconomic status. My mother seized the opportunity to reinforce her favorite mantra, "In this world, you will need to be twice as good to get half as far as people who do not look like you." Instead of relying on my counselor to lead me through the college process, my mother, who only has an 8th grade education, went to the only person she knew who understood the process. She scheduled a meeting with my pediatrician. You see, in our neighborhood, we were lucky enough to have both an African American Dentist and Pediatrician.

Dr. Williams was a warm and gentle soul who never rushed when seeing his patients and never turned you away for lack of payment. He scheduled a meeting with my mother and I and offered advice, guidance and financial support. Because of his generosity and altruism, I received scholarships from four different local black organizations. With this money and grants, I was able to pay my college tuition. This selfless act of giving was my first experience of receiving a helping hand from someone who was genuinely interested in my success. Dr. Williams understood his role in our community included helping others less fortunate to achieve goals. Before Affirmative Action, this was the standard in my community. Each One Teach One is an African-American proverb dating back to slavery; it is embedded in our culture to remind us we have a responsibility to educate and help others because the color of our skin limits the opportunities available to us. He taught me it would take 3-5 generations to hardwire education as a tool to eradicate poverty. I embraced being at ground zero as the first person in my family to attend college. It meant failure wasn't an option and generations that weren't even born yet depended on my success. This was a heavy load to carry, but I was enthusiastic about the challenge.

My college years continued to offer me experiences that shaped my career and the person I am today. At one point, I faced a challenge regarding one of my scholarships. In my junior year, I decided to pledge an African-American Greek sorority. As I researched the sororities on my campus, many students told me that the dark berry color of my skin meant I had to pledge the red sorority because I was too dark to pledge the pink one. This was a pivotal point in my college career. No way would I accept discrimination within my own race. Needless to say I pledged the pink and lost my scholarship from the red, which I had not even considered as a possibility. But, as my mother often said, "what doesn't kill you will make you stronger." This situation forced me to multitask in a new way. The next semester, I took a full load at the University and 6 additional units at the Junior College. I also worked 3 jobs and did this using public transportation. My commitment to college never wavered because of the financial set back. Instead, it made me more determined to finish college and I vowed to never depend on anyone for anything.

Although I was hurt and very disappointed after I met with the African-American medical doctor who told me they would no longer honor my scholarship, I sort of understood their position in not wanting to provide financial support to the rival sorority. I remember the tears I shed as I left her office and the feeling of disgust and shock at the vast difference in her attitude and commitment towards my college education from that of Dr. Williams, my pediatrician. I had incorrectly assumed that all African-American successful people embraced the role of Each One Teach One. This one episode was instrumental in shaping my purpose in life.

It's important to remember that every person you meet has a story that is uniquely theirs and has powerfully shaped their life. Understanding a person's past will help you embrace their current position.

I started the nursing program in the fall of 1985, the same year that I got married. We lived 2 hours away from campus near the Air Force Base where my husband was stationed. Every day, I braved the crazy commuter traffic in the Bay Area driving a car without air or heat in hopes of making it to class on time. I got pregnant the first year of the nursing program. My stomach grew so large that I was unable to fit behind the wheel of my little car. My brothers, who were so proud of me for going to college, helped out by taking turns driving me to school. On one occasion, my brother, the drug dealer, hired a cab to take me and bring me home. This is the same brother who would send a mechanic to fix my car on the side of the freeway after I broke down headed to class and the same brother who taught me the value of reading and education. He was my biggest supporter. He is incarcerated now for drug related charges and I have spent the last 20 years paying back this debt by loving and supporting him. No matter where he is, I visit regularly. My success is in part due to his support and encouragement.

I delivered my beautiful baby boy just two days after Christmas 1986, and four weeks later I was back in school with a newborn in tow. I spent the next 2 years struggling through nursing school with a baby. I took him to all my lectures and sat in the back of the class with him taking notes and trying to keep him quiet. Some days I sat outside in the hallway with the door cracked, listening to the lecture and watching him play at the same time. There were students in my cohort that were very supportive. When it was time to take exams, we would split the two-hour block of time. They would try to finish in an hour so one of them could watch my son while I went in to take the exam. Caring for a small child, commuting 2 hours to school, working 2 part time jobs and going to school full time took a toll and one day while driving to my practicum assignment, I blanked out on where I was and where I was going. I pulled over on the side of the

Chapter 4

freeway and began crying uncontrollably. A highway patrol officer stopped to find out if I needed help. He called my father and waited the 2 hours with me until my family arrived to take me home. This wasn't the first concerning incident I had. A few weeks earlier, I was driving home from school and was a few miles from my home exit when I was pulled over by a cop with lights and siren. He explained he had been following me for 2 miles with his lights on and I didn't pull over. He was pulling me over because I was driving too slowly. I was so exhausted that I was numb and unaware of my surroundings. I suspect I was basically asleep with my eyes open. The two incidents forced me to take a semester off from school to regroup. Even this did not deter me from completing college. I completed the program, studied hard and passed the NCLEX on my first try.

Growth and Development

Throughout my nursing career and young adulthood, I enjoyed success and failures that defined me as a person and leader. As a novice nurse a few years into my career, my biological father died. Not the father who raised me since I was 2 years old, but the one responsible for my being born. My siblings and I, five in total, along with my 3½-year-old son, traveled by van from California to Missouri to bury my father. Although we had limited interactions with him over the years, we all felt a sense of responsibility to attend his funeral. On the way back from Missouri we encountered a snowstorm in Colorado that yielded black ice on the roads. My family was in a terrible car accident that left a toddler dead, massive injuries to all involved. Except me. Although I was thrown from the vehicle, I landed on my knees in the middle of the freeway and suffered only minor bruises. The rest of my family survived but suffered horrible injuries. My eldest brother was driving and had the entire dashboard and steering wheel in his chest. My youngest brother's head went through the windshield landing inches from the big rig that we slammed into. He broke his neck and was placed in a halo to stabilize his neck. My son broke both femurs and was in a body cast for months. My sister and other brother both suffered multiple broken bones and had casted extremities. The mental scars from that event continue to affect me today. However, that one event restored my faith in a higher power. My family was able to fly home only if a nurse accompanied them. I firmly believe I was spared serious injury because it was my role to ensure my small tribe of the walking wounded made it home safely. When we boarded the plane, I was proud to produce my nursing license to provide proof of my abilities to escort my family home. This experience was humbling, as it tested my ability to perform under pressure, and it reminded me there is a higher power.

Another experience that impacted my growth as a nurse leader happened about 7 years into my career, when a position for Assistant Nurse Manager became available. I recall sitting in the break room as my peers pointed each other out and encouraged each other to apply for the position. I took note that none of them encouraged me to apply. I was instantly transported back to my college days when I was told I couldn't pledge a certain sorority. That evening, I told my mom about the incident. True to who she is, she reminded me that I could do anything I wanted to do. The next day I applied for the position. Needless to say it was a shock to the entire staff when I was selected for the position. My manager saw my leadership abilities as well as my desire to fix everyone's problems. She was the first person in my professional life to encourage me to own only those things that I should own. She was my first mentor and coach. She was honest, straight to the point and very professional. Her feedback and mentorship helped me identify my strengths and weaknesses. The one lesson that I never forgot was to set myself for success by developing a strong independent high functioning team, a team that did not require me to hold them up but to hold them together. A very powerful lesson.

Daily Affirmation

I read somewhere that a strong woman is the lifeline of her family. She carries within her the power to endure pain and the courage to sacrifice. She has the power to create and nurture life. She is, indeed, the epitome of love and sacrifice. Every day I am reminded of the lives I've touched and the difference I have made - from family members that I took in and raised to nurses that I have mentored and patients that I have cared for. These daily affirmations keep me fighting to make a difference in my work and private life. But these things are not enough to hold me up and support my well-being. That I have to do on my own. As a caretaker, it is much more comfortable to care for others than yourself.

Courage and Strength

For the majority of my life I focused on caring for others. At work, I was paid to care for patients; at home, I cared for my immediate and extended family. When my son left for college, I went through the normal mid-life crisis from being an empty nester. I, like so many other women, had built a life around being a mother and wife. And like other mid-life crisis women, I needed to re-direct my energy to a different cause - so I bought a Harley-Davidson and left my job of 17 years in search of something more challenging. When I shared with my neighbors my plan to relocate to a new city for work, they were less shocked about the motorcycle and job change than they were to learn we only had 1 child. You see, for the better part of ten years, we had parented in our home so many nieces and nephews, the neighbors assumed we had several children. When I mentioned this to my son some years later he said, "Mom, I can only remember maybe one school year or a partial year that I went to school without one of my cousins." My commitment to my family and my passion for nurturing and caring for others had become my purpose in life for the last 20 years.

Buying my Harley Davidson motorcycle was the first action in my entire life that I did simply because I wanted to. Against my husband's advice, I bought a brand new 2005 Softail Deluxe, 6 months after my son left for college. At 43 years of age, it was my first act of self-care.

Self-care is defined in many ways. In health care, it is any necessary human regulatory function, which is under individual control, which is deliberate and self-initiated. We know from research a lack of self-care can lead to burnout in certain professions, such as social work and nursing. Burnout is a combination of mental, emotional and physical exhaustion. Therefore, self-care is crucial for our mental, emotional and physical well-being. Some people engage in meditation, exercise, behavioral therapy and any other number of activities to meet their spiritual, physical and emotional self-care needs. Unfortunately, none of this worked for me. I am my most happiest when I am doing for others - my emotional self-care needs are easily met through work and caring for my family. As a nurse, I am well aware this is not a healthy state to exist in. Health care is full of professionals who lack the ability to care for themselves, and this can and will lead to burnout. The challenge is with identifying your own needs and taking the necessary steps to meet them. But how do you take time away from caring for others to care for yourself? For some of us this is a difficult task; treating yourself as kindly as you treat others is a conscious deliberate act that requires self-reflection, insight and planning.

As I mentioned earlier in this chapter, my first act of self-care involved throwing caution to the wind and doing something just because I wanted to. It was non-traditional and totally out of character for me to buy a motorcycle. I didn't know how to ride a motorcycle and didn't know anyone who rode a motorcycle. But it satisfied my growing desire to do something for myself that was not connected to who I was and how people saw me. I was growing tired of being the responsible person who did everything by the book; the dependable, stable one. I wanted to find a different path for self-care that was not connected to caring for others. Interestingly, within a few months of my motorcycle purchase, three of my brothers, a sister, my husband and son, as well as my niece and several cousins, all bought motorcycles as well. Within a year we were a motorcycle family of a dozen or more. Through this process I discovered a totally different type of inner strength that changed my self-care trajectory. I began to understand self-care is not always isolated from caring for others; that for some of us, it is a blended process where one action compliments and supports the other. For those of us who have a strong need to do for others, we have to explore our own feelings to determine why this act of giving is so gratifying and what role it plays in our self-worth.

Self-Reflection

When I reflect back on my childhood, I clearly remember being different from my 3 sisters. My eldest sister was the beautiful one. She was caramel colored, tall and thin and began a modeling career in high school. My youngest sister…well…she was the baby in the family - who can compete with that? My sister just under me had the crown jewel of my community: beautiful long, thick, black hair and the biggest, prettiest eyes. And then there was me. I was practically bald through my toddler years, with a very dark black skin tone. If long pretty hair was the crown jewel in my community, being of very dark skin tone was the curse - an automatic description of ugly. Thankfully, I was raised by one of the smartest mothers around. She knew the importance of instilling confidence in her girls, and, from an early age, I was praised for my intelligence and wit. So I was the smart one. I wore this as a badge of honor, because as the elders in my community were quick to say, "Beauty is only skin deep and will fade over time; brains are lifelong." Being smart gave me an edge because it meant my siblings came to me, the smart one, to help them figure out problems. Even my mother and father enlisted my assistance, from a very early age, with helping them to read and understand official documents. I became the go to person in my family for issue resolutions and it felt good. It validated my importance in the family and solidified my caretaker role.

This role also required me to speak for my family members and fight the battles of those that weren't strong enough. I'm reminded of the time when my baby sister got a new job but was too scared to quit her current job. I stepped in and quit her job for her by calling the owner of the dental practice and explaining her position. When the job didn't work out, I again stepped in and got her the old job back. I have stepped in to resolve issues that family and friends have been unable to solve. I can recall the powerful feeling of accomplishment and the exhilaration of knowing I could get things done that others couldn't. These are the feelings that validated my self-worth and kept me on the path of caring for others while ignoring my own self-care needs.

Self-Discovery

It was during my first year of riding a motorcycle that I discovered my need to be a caretaker was a problem. Within a few months of riding, I met a group of other professional black women who all road Harleys. Together we became the Road Queens MC. One of the members was an airline pilot named Fly Girl who became my unofficial big sister. In many ways we were alike, in that we had strong personalities and we were used to being in charge. We shared another quality that I was not accustomed to seeing in anyone else in my circle. She was also a caretaker of sorts, as she is generally the one in her circle that makes the decisions, cares for family members and shoulders financial responsibilities. For the first time in my life, I had someone who looked out for me, bought me things or paid my way and made decisions without my input. She called me her little sister, and regardless of where we rode - Arizona, Nevada or across country - she tried to take care of me. In the beginning, I struggled with this. I thought it was a reflection of my ability to care for myself, or it spoke to my riding ability. Finally one day she asked why I was quick to do for others but didn't want people to do for me. After careful consideration and reflection I realized by having people do things for me took away the exhilarating feelings I got when I do for others. It triggered feelings of neediness and weakness rather than how I saw myself as strong, independent and self-assured. It took years for me to allow and accept acts of kindness from others. I was so accustomed to being the giver, receiving was a foreign concept that I, in part, didn't want because it threatened my feelings of power and control. Over time, I learned to redefine how to care for others while

Chapter 4

caring for myself. Allowing for a marrying of the two concepts sometimes created conflict, but most often they co-existed due to the lessons learned over years of maturation, growth and development.

Self-Care

My self-care lessons are rooted not in the traditional sense of self-care such as meditation or exercise; rather, they are rooted in the fight or flight response; a physiological reaction that occurs in response to a perceived threat. My culture and upbringing has predisposed me to certain feelings of inadequacy and injustice. This threat of inadequacy has driven me to become a successful Nurse Executive, but it has also made me neglect caring for myself as I fought battles and cared for others. Through experiences, I have developed some techniques that have proven to assist me on my journey.

- Years ago, I realized I needed to define who I was as a leader and what I aimed to accomplish. I had to embrace the fighter spirit, yet tame the delivery of my words. This self-care helped to decrease anxiety in situations that required a crucial conversation. It allowed me to stand up for others and feed my inner need while taking care of myself at the same time

- Recognizing and embracing who you are allows you to be your most authentic self. Instead of trying to change how I was seen by others - aggressive, overbearing, self-assured, loud - I embraced these qualities and openly discussed them with other executives and staff. Not to apologize for my behavior, but to explain my leadership style and the benefits of the frank, open conversations it supported. By doing this upfront, others and I could accept my differences as the diversity an organization needs to perform and produce at the highest level.

- Motivating self and others through visionary leadership and real talk. Creating a culture of acceptance is key to a successful team and is contagious among team members. I aim to leave a legacy of acceptance at work and in my community. Hearing from people that I have inspired and motivated is a form of self-care because I know my work will live on.

- Gifting of yourself every day to others and yourself. I truly believe when you gift something of yourself it helps you to be a better person. Every day I try to gift myself something of value. It could be time to grieve a loss or time to sit quietly in contemplation of my blessing. Sometimes it is as small as a 15 extra minutes under a hot shower or as big as a full on spa day. When I got pregnant with my son, my mother sat me down and explained that the next 18 years of my life belonged to my child, but to never stop taking care of myself. I was in my 40s before I realized what she meant. Having something that is uniquely yours, and yours alone, is a form of self-care because the only opinion that matters is yours.

- Be SEX-C. Set an Example of Xtradinary; you choose the C. Some days its Compassion, Caring or Communication. Depending on the situation, I have to remind myself that I have the ability to be extraordinary in all that I do. My C is often Calm, Colorful, Creative, Careful, Collaboration and Caring. These words are a part of my personal mantra to carefully remain calm in my colorful delivery of creative collaboration to care for you and me. It is my way of accepting and embracing that my view of self-care is closely linked to caring for others.

- Understanding and accepting the environment in which you live and work. Self-care in this form gives you permission to pick and choose your battles with the knowledge that some situations will require you to tackle head on, while others simply require a savviness to maneuver around. When you relinquish ownership of problems or issues that are not your own, you engage in self-care.

- Live life to its fullest, outside of your comfort zone and be adventurous. These things will expose you to different worldviews and encourage a new level of acceptance of others. This self-care removes limits on your thinking and forces you to compare and contrast your values with the values of others.

- Identify triggers that cause you anxiety. When you know the things that upset your internal balance, you can work toward decreasing or eliminating the triggers.

- Build into your day those things that bring you joy. It is the simple things in life, like the laughter of your grandchild, or the wind in your face as you peel down the highway on your bike, that are the best measures of self-care. They remind you of your blessings and of how far you have traveled on your journey.

End of the Road

My passion to care for others started when I was a child, caring for neighborhood kids and my younger siblings, progressed through high school, when I would speak out against injustices, and stayed with me through adulthood as I rallied for those who were weaker and afraid to fight for themselves. I am a born caretaker and I embrace this role. My journey was rough and took longer than I expected. I have had medical setbacks that resulted in 4 surgeries in the last 6 years. This has not stopped me from doing the things I enjoy and continuing to work in the profession I love - nursing. It was during this time that I reflected on how the lack of self-care may have contributed to my medical issues.

I have reached the top position in my profession and I am comfortable in my family/home life. For the last 5 years, my self-care has centered on monthly time-outs. Every month I take a few days off from work and travel to a relaxing place that soothes my soul. Sometimes it's a simple weekend get-away; other times it's a full week resort stay. Whatever I do, I am careful to spend this time rejuvenating and caring for my soul. Through my 40 year journey, I have learned valuable lessons that shaped and molded me into a passionate, patient advocate, a fierce nursing leader, a compassionate caretaker and a strong black woman with a zest for living life to its fullest and never allowing adversities to defeat me.

About The Author

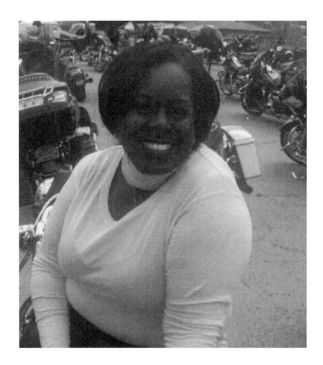

Barbara Barney-Knox is a Chief Nurse Executive for California Correctional Health Care Services (CCHCS). She is responsible for the oversight of nurse professional practice and compliance throughout the 35 prisons in California. In this capacity, Barbara and her team of Nurse Consultant Program Reviewers work collaboratively with institutions to identify clinical practice departures and best practices that may have an impact on patient care. Barbara has been with CCHCS for 4 years and has been instrumental in developing and implementing Shared Governance, a nursing professional practice model that empowers nurses to have a voice in decisions that impact nursing.

Prior to working for CCHCS, Barbara spent 8 years as a leader at Kaiser Permanente and 17 years at the University of California

Davis Health System. Barbara received her BSN from San Jose State University almost 30 years ago. She has a Masters in Psychology and recently graduated Summa Cum Laude with her MBA.

As a leader, Barbara has accumulated awards and accolades throughout her career. She is the 2010 recipient of the Nurse of Distinction Award from Chi Eta Tau Nursing Sorority and has also received several awards from the University of California Davis, including the Nurse Excellence Award, the Ambassador of Diversity Award and Manager of the Year Award for receiving Patient Satisfaction Scores in the 95th percentile for 4 consecutive quarters. Other recognitions include Kaiser Permanente Work Place Safety Award for Injury and Illness Prevention and a nomination for the American Nurses Association National Nurse of Excellence Award.

In her career Barbara has been selected to present at several professional conferences, including the American Nurses Credentialing Center (ANCC), the National Magnet Conference, ANCC Med/Surg Conference and the CA/NV American Correctional Health Services Association Annual Conference.

In her spare time, Barbara is a motorcycle enthusiast and has rode across country on her Harley Davidson on four occasions.

Contact Information:

Email: ebonyrider13@gmail.com
Email: Barbara.barney-knox@cdcr.ca.gov

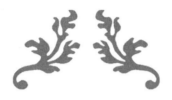

CHAPTER 5

When I Found My Voice

My mother was fourteen years old and my father was sixteen years old when I was born. They were too young to know about parenting, but old enough to become parents. Both were wild and free, without a care in the world, living with my grandmother in the Oakland, California projects. But, with all of this free living came responsibility. I needed to be taken care of, fed and clothed. After taking me to friends and family so that they could party and hang out, my parents ultimately left me with Doll and James, my Godparents.

James and Doll had no children together, so they went to my mother and asked if they could help take care of me by buying my clothes and any other necessities I needed. Of course, my parents said ok. Why not? Besides, they had no money to take care of me. James and Doll taught me about traveling as a young girl. We fished, went to concerts, swam in the local rivers and did everything a little girl could imagine. At the age of two months, I started staying with them on the weekends, leading to weekdays, to ultimately living with them full time in the sixth grade. James was retired military, and from the time I can remember, he was very disciplined, very organized and he loved numbers. With only a sixth-grade education, he prided himself on understanding his paycheck and calculating it prior to picking it up. From the time I was six years old, he had me sit opposite him at the kitchen table while I read a book or did my homework and learned how to count money. I had to be quiet and speak when spoken to. I carried this with me through high school. In my 8th grade year, James told me

Chapter 5

he thought I should be a nurse. But, who wants to do what their parents wanted? Not me...

On the other hand, my mother was the first in the family to go to college, but she later had a problem with drugs, which she overcame later in life. She was nurturing, fun, loved people and loved taking care of others. I can remember times when she picked me up after getting paid, and cashing her check at the check cashing place and handing me a wad of money from her purse. She gave handfuls of money to everyone, never counting what she gave them.

This is where my story begins...

As I look back now, the nurse in me came from my mother, as I inherited her traits as a nurturer, and the business side of me came from my godfather, as a man who paid attention to his money. I was my own version of the story *Rich Dad, Poor Dad*, meaning I learned how to manage money early (becoming an entrepreneur) and learning how to work hard doing what I loved - helping people (becoming a nurse).

James and Doll started preparing me for college in the third grade, and when I reached 12th grade, I applied to three large universities and was accepted to all of them. It helped that I had a 3.98 GPA. I chose UC Davis, with a major in pre-med. Yes, I thought I wanted to become a doctor. Between my timidity and the shock of coming from an ill-prepared school from Oakland, California into a huge university like UC Davis, I was not prepared for the rigorous curriculum. I received my first "F" in biology at this school. Devastated and homesick, I tried to go home, but James wasn't having it. They moved into a 1-bedroom house with a sofa bed not allowing me a place to return. After I received the "F," I changed my major to dietetics and learned how to move around in college. I graduated, but I knew I was missing something and shortly got my first job as a dietician. That job was not what I thought. As a dietician, my office was in the kitchen. I would see patients for their dietary needs and end up sitting on their beds, getting them water, or just talking to them. I realized I did want to be a nurse. James was right, so I prepared myself for the journey to nursing school. At that time, I was a single mother and dirt poor. I applied to nursing school and was rejected. Finally, the Friday before the Monday of the first day of nursing school, I got the call saying I was accepted. I had been doing odd jobs waiting for acceptance and eagerly told them I was quitting the next day. I had no money saved but went as if I did. I found twelve scholarships totaling $7,500 and completed nursing school with honors.

It was my last semester of nursing school when I got the news that my mother was in the hospital and to come now. She was 47 years old. I entered the ER when the doctor pulled me to the side to try and prepare me for what I was about to see. I entered the room to find a tube in her mouth, she was not moving, and a white sheet covered her body. She was dead…she had a massive heart attack. I went numb.

As time went by, I tried to bury the emotions of mourning my mother by telling myself to think about the ordeal later. This worked until it came time to take my nursing boards. I arrived at the location only to have a panic attack 10 minutes into the test. My mother's face appeared on the computer screen, smiling as

Chapter 5

she looked directly at me. I did not pass the test. I couldn't get past her face. This happened 2 more times before I realized I needed to deal with my emotions. So, I took some time off, went away alone, prayed, read and relished any good memory I had with my mother until I could feel her in my heart again. I realized I was angry at her for giving me away, but in theory, giving me away prepared me for who I am today. As for the nursing boards…the 3rd time did it; I passed. I knew then that I wanted to be a cardiac nurse.

Nursing became my passion, I yearned to learn all I could about nursing by rotating through all the professions: orthopedic, neurology, oncology, telemetry, surgery, recovery and many more. But, I always came back to telemetry. I wanted my patients to get resolution from their heart issues before they had trouble and could potentially have a heart attack like my mother. As I taught patients the importance of diet, why they needed to stop doing drugs and how to balance medication, my confidence grew. My voice became solid, strong and tenacious, unlike the meek, insecure voice I always had because I was afraid others would think I was smart. Yes, I said it - "I am smart" and I'm ok with it.

Time passed, and I soon wanted more. I begin taking tax classes and became a tax preparer. I felt like I woke up the gentle giant in me. I wanted even more. Anything that had to do with numbers, I wanted to know about it. I finally decided to return to school and get my MBA in finance. I had watched my fellow nurses work hard, making $200-$300 thousand dollars a year and have nothing to show for it. They knew nothing about their money. They took care of everyone else but not themselves. MiKash Corporation was born. It became my passion to teach every nurse, man, or woman I knew and didn't know about their money and educating them on financial literacy. I had arrived. I can now do what my heart desires, taking care of others medically and taking care of those who take care of others - my fellow nurses. This leads into how I can continue being a nurse and an entrepreneur. I gear these careers with the same tenacity and strength today as I did twenty-four years ago.

Seasoned nurses know that new nurses will soon realize that nursing is not an easy job, nor is it for everyone. However, it is self-fulfilling, selfless and a work of art painted on the heart of every patient touched with gentleness, kindness, joy and love. Giving to others is a commandment of God, but what you get in return is limitless. Everyone has a story and every story has an ending, but if you decide to choose your destiny with a goal in mind, then you will write your legacy and live it the way you want.

Self-Love, Self-Discipline, Self-Respect

The main way I choose to take care of myself is by routine maintenance for my spirit, body and mind. I love me more than anyone else can, other than my father in heaven.

To give others any part of who I am as a person, a woman, a mother, a grandmother, a nurse, or a businesswoman, I must take care of me first and foremost. I achieve this through self-discipline, self-love and self-respect.

I am an acute care telemetry nurse. My patients are acutely ill. They have come to the hospital unwillingly, some unknowingly, and most are not themselves. They feel bad and their normal routine is gone. We take their clothes, give them our rules, tell them when to eat, brush their teeth and even when to walk. So, when I walk into a room of a patient I have never met, with minimal information as to why they are in the hospital, I need to have all my faculties. My mind should be clear and on task to the situation in front of me. I should be prepared for the worse on every entry into a patient's room. Knowing that the unimaginable could happen could lead to a level of distress if I allowed myself to focus on it. But I don't. I've learned to accept this unknown expectation with the understanding that my background and knowledge base can guide me through any situation. This includes acknowledging and accepting all available resources. I call this thought process the resource bin of my mind.

The ability to tolerate discomfort is a requirement for raising my personal standard, sometimes… What type of discomfort you may ask? The discomfort of understanding that I cannot fix everything or everyone. The discomfort of toleration of things that are intolerable. The discomfort of rejection from others who have no relevance to me being who I am. I choose daily to understand that I did not wake myself up this morning or any morning. That I trust in the power of God and that discomfort is a thorn that needs to be plucked and discarded if it affects me being the best I can be. Or, in some cases, tolerating a form of discomfort necessary to take me to the next level in my personal growth.

Choose not to neglect yourself. Choose to love you first. Choose to listen to that inner voice of rationality. Choose to take care of yourself so that you can take care of others. This is what we, as nurses, chose to do. Don't let the dirty footsteps of other's chaos and misfortune walk through your thoughts.

My self-love routine is simple. I work hard and I play hard. I have enough vacation time to take a good vacation and still have enough remaining for an emergency. I take a minimum of 4 vacations a year; one alone with me, myself, and I (all at one time), one with my family, one with my man and one with all of us together. Not using vacation is a misfortune to you and your patients because vacations allow you to rejuvenate your mind, body and soul. It allows you to disconnect from the burden of worry - for your patients, family, or friends - that nurses carry. The ability to relax your mind from the barrage of policies and protocols is necessary to perform your job. Spending time with your personal, long-time friends, as well as like-minded professional friends, is also important. Friends on both parameters encourage your personal growth, as well as offer availability for times of comfort. Other things, such as reading, exercising, eating right, weight management, yoga, etc. are objectives that are carved into your self-love journey as well.

Self-discipline is the foundation of understanding why we as nurses and individuals need to take care of ourselves. Because without discipline to hold yourself accountable to the priceless duties entrusted to you as a person, mother, father, nurse, or any profession held, you could not perform those duties. Disciplines, such as arriving to work on time and with a good attitude (which can dictate your patient's care), reading assigned emails, completing education prerequisites on time and keeping up with immunizations, are to name a few. Knowing what you are responsible for and following through on what you need to do is a discipline that cannot be taken away from you, both personally and professionally.

Finally, self-respect. Respect yourself first and foremost. Know your tolerance and acceptance of situations and stand by it. I choose to respect myself by allowing different assumptions to lead to different choices when necessary. By allowing situations, good or bad, to result in an opportunity for growth is healthy for me personally. Personal growth is exciting and exuberating, but can be painful and exhausting at times. But, it is necessary for wholeness, because as I stated earlier, I love me some me....I respect me for being me, beautifully made, whole, healthy, with a heart for people. Understand, there really are people who do not innately have a natural tendency to help others; they must work at it. As a nurse, with any level of self-respect, it is important to have this trait, to nourish it and encompass it so that you never lose it.

About Author

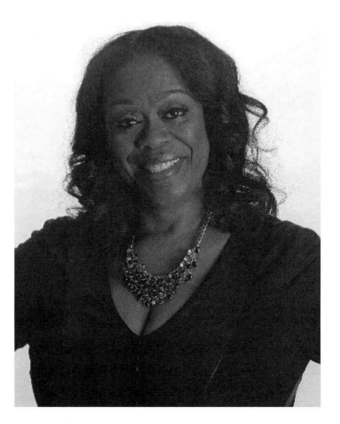

Donna Rosby AA, RN, BS, MBA is a registered nurse, book author, entrepreneur, investor and businesswoman. Born and raised in Oakland, California, she initially started her career working as a dietician for one year before starting nursing school some years later. Donna has worked in all areas of nursing, with the last eight years as a bedside cardiac nurse for two different prominent northern California hospitals, simultaneously. While working as a nurse, she self-studied the stock market, which has encouraged her to share her knowledge with fellow nurses by starting a stock club. The success of the stock club has prompted her to open other clubs with family and friends and assist others in opening their own investment clubs. Donna is now the President of multiple investment clubs that aim to educate and empower both nurses and others to become financially independent via the stock market and other investment vehicles.

While working as a nurse, Donna completed her MBA in Finance, after which she started her own company, Mikash Corporation. Her company focuses on financial literacy by offering multiple forms of financial education for nurses and others. Some of Donna's specialties are: budget preparation, retirement planning, tax preparation, annuities, insurance, 401k/IRA assistance, asset allocation, credit repair and a specialty in the initiation of stock club(s) for nurses and individuals. As Donna's business continues to progress, she continues to expand her products by adding books, workbooks and journals. Donna has completed a children's finance book, with a children's nursing book in progress, and adult finance books to follow.

To Contact the Author:

President/CEO MiKash Corporation
Email: Donna@mikash.net
Website: mikash.net

CHAPTER 6

The Calling

I'm standing at my grandfather's bed, making sure he doesn't fall, as only half of his body is actually functional. He is attempting to relieve himself and I am pretending that I am anywhere but there. I'm twelve years old. Assisting my grandfather with this sort of support, because of his debilitating stroke, was my earliest introduction to what it means to be a nurse. Since that time, I have encountered a multitude of experiences of what it entails to be apart of the wonderful complexities that make up the field of nursing. Nursing in its wisdom has the ability to both humble and lift you. Nursing delivers its true practitioners into a more authentic, more mentally and emotionally intelligent and more spiritual space than I think any other Calling can do.

I remember I started telling people that I wanted to be a nurse before it was actually "cool" for men to be nurses. Perhaps it was sitting wide eyed and intrigued, watching the early seasons of "ER" that started me on this way, or perhaps those little plastic doctor kits I used to play with as a child, that had a fake stethoscope and some band-aids, that sparked the interest of claiming nursing as apart of my identity. More substantially, my soul sensed a call that continually knocked at my inner door, asking if I would answer. Even a child can be intuitive enough to respond to the quiet Calling, and in hearing ones "yes," life begins to send "icons" to encourage you, to redirect you and to establish you in its own quiet and powerful way towards that fulfilling journey.

Once the Call is clearly distinguished, there will be a sense of "duty" to see the Calling manifested in a more realistic way.

Chapter 6

Prerequisite courses, nursing school and all the qualifications to operate dynamically as "nurse" will need a refining discipline in order to sift away the part of us that refuses to arise and grow, that part of us that refuses to be a true learner. Discipline is your champion now because passion is not yet stable. In my own journey, I learned that passion to be a nurse didn't serve me as much as discipline did. Passion will bring excitement and expose how intimate you want to be with your calling, but discipline will fortify the foundation to build that career, and foundation is everything. Once discipline to maintain your course is established, passion can then enter back in and operate as a wind to the sails.

I think that for every true Calling that comes to us, the part of us that I call the "non-learner" attempts to hang you up. The non-learner is the opposing force to all the things that aspire to grow in and out of us. I must warn you, the non-learner part of us is never truly banished, even by discipline. The non-learner is a chronic non-participator. The non-learner is lazy, the non-learner is disinterested, the non-learner is unmotivated, and be careful, because the non-learner part of us seems to get some sort of twisted satisfaction when it becomes the primary driver of our lives, always leading in the opposite direction of our dream, or worse, locking us in the "imagination station" of our dream instead of the actual experience of it. The non-learner whispers, "I'm too busy, I have other people I have to take care of." The non-participatory, non-learner part of our mentalities operates in an element of cowardice towards the truth, which is that a powerful and very capable person wants to sprout out from the middle of no-where. But I encourage you to let your no-where be your now-here!

I recall aspiring to be a nurse for many years before I felt and saw true results. It was as if it was all up-hill for a while, and even simple hiking trails seemed, at times, like Mt. Everest. I swear it took me one-hundred years and one-thousand attempts at passing certain math and chemistry classes that were required in order to get accepted into the nursing program. I became discouraged and my mind told me I would never succeed, that I wasn't cut out to be smart or to be an academic achiever. But that voice was not speaking the truest truth and the best thing I have ever done in my life was learn to abandon the influence of the non-learner.

Many nurses tell me that nursing is a career where you continually learn for the entirety of the experience. This knowing that "no one knows all things about everything" is a good nursing sensibility. My advice is to learn this before you even get the nursing degree! This knowing that you don't know and can't know everything sprouts out of the necessary humility it takes to get the job done. This humility is vital to the nursing foundation that allows you the opportunity to be a quality learner and offers the necessary pliability to make room for the human experience within the job.

It is in the humble and authentic choosing to stay a learner that something of significance takes place, intellectual competence and emotional intelligence can unionize. Intellectual competence and emotional intelligence are two forests whose roots run deep into the field of nursing. Their roots take to the soil, and underneath, in an unseen place, they meet together, fortifying what lies above the soil - you. I recall my first nursing instructor explaining this as,

Chapter 6

"Nursing is an art and a science and you will need both to be a good nurse."

Anyone who passes the threshold that is nursing school knows that you leave a part of you behind…but this person left behind is not a part of you that is truly you, only a part that you thought was you. I remember waking up at four-thirty in the morning and being introduced to the discipline required to accomplish nursing school. No one understands the struggle and the energy it takes to resist exiting at the nearest exit of Comfort and Complacency. But don't fear, though the learning and refining process will appear lonely at times. Life will send companions to lighten the load. Like a group of disciples giving themselves to the discipline, the camaraderie generates enough enduring power to get to the next destination. Likely these will be nursing or aspiring nursing students who, upon fellowship, seem to kindle your own drive to see the dream become a reality. The day in and day out of this experience begins to reveal in you the ability to see farther, work harder and to take more accountability for the entire process.

The pathway of obtaining your nursing degree can be long and arduous and it will be necessary to drive this path utilizing the correct fuel in your tank. This pathway is a cross country one and having a powerful source of motivation will be required if you are to succeed. I have always found it a bit humorous when people need "haters" in order to be empowered to accomplish a goal. To me it's like eating a candy bar before a work out as opposed to a protein bar - it won't last you and actually works against you. I'm not saying it can't be a source of fuel for a rapid sprint or a foothold to hoist you over an obstacle, but my point is that it operates on a lower spiritual frequency. I would encourage you to find a more wholesome source of motivation. I would suggest utilizing your own internal power that is offered from your soul, as it offers a greater satisfaction and leaves your spirit feeling light and your mind less crowded.

Those that see the process as a race, or a battle against others, actually reveal an internal struggle indicating a damaged relationship with their own selves. This competitive spirit does not have a place in the heart of nursing, and nurses and aspiring nurses who operate in this way often struggle with self worth, depression and inclusion with the team, and nursing is ALL about the team! The reality is that there is another source of power we can tap into as nurses. There is a greater sense of purpose to just be that which you are called to be that gently motivates the current that pushes you towards accomplishment.

It takes a quiet and reflective mind to allow this energy to offer its natural and nutritional motivation for the journey. I call this "The Spirituality of the Health Care Worker." This spirituality is present across health care workers and many who offer their energy in service to others. The aroma that is produced when operating in the maturity of one who serves others is kindness, patience, advocacy and love. Even the gruffest of individuals can operate in this light when they maintain the course within their spiritual calling to serve others.

On the "journey to becoming," the mind is literally undergoing reconstruction. The learning of new facts can literally change the tissue within the brain! This is evidence that spiritual callings can manifest in the physical, and you will see the evidence as your

Chapter 6

mind exceeds its previous capabilities again and again. After awhile, you will see that it is this "tide" of moving forward and going back, moving forward and going back, that becomes the actual destination. Ride this tide; participate by allowing this spirituality to mature you into a wave rider! Its waves will take you in and out of peoples lives, healing, touching, speaking, singing, laughing, crying and experiencing the wonder of the human condition.

The human condition is a remarkable one, absolutely remarkable. Very early within the journey of "becoming" that one element of the human condition that all humans seek to avoid will present itself to you in order to check your authenticity. That element is human suffering. The only reason the role or the ministry of nursing exists within the human condition is because of human suffering. Do you know how you will respond when human suffering presents itself?

I often "hear" the response from people when they find out I am a nurse, and it goes something like this, "Thank you so much for being a nurse; I definitely couldn't do that, especially since I can't stand the sight of blood." Sure, there are some people who literally cannot stand the sight of blood (though somehow they can watch hundreds of movies that have bloody content), but what I am really "hearing" is their confession that they cannot stand comfortably within the presence of human suffering. It is only by the presence of human suffering that the role of nursing exists. Not all nurses need to be trauma or ER nurses but all effective nurses will have, at some point, learned to stand in the presence of human suffering and offer an opposing light to that sorrowful darkness.

How you will allow this encounter to change you will determine your effectiveness as a health care practitioner. If the ministry of "nurse" awakens within you and you find a compelling urgency to alleviate that suffering, then you know you are on the correct course. I recall my first week at the bedside. I was working in physical therapy at that time and was assisting a physical therapist with a patient that had a debilitating stroke. The patient was a Latin man in his late 60s. When I looked at him, for some reason he reminded me and, strangely enough, looked exactly like my grandfather. I was stunned. I stared at him while he unsuccessfully attempted to roll to the side of the bed. Being trapped within your own body while it refuses to work is a unique type of human suffering. As I stared at him, I could sense that my vision was closing in. I felt faint. I stabled myself against the bed and I acutely recall thinking to myself, "Can I do this?"

This was the Calling introducing me to my discomfort with human suffering. I took a deep breath and assisted the physical therapist with helping this gentleman to sit upright. Helping another human being to regain their function and dignity when they cannot do so for themselves requires that you resolve your discomfort with human suffering. Human suffering is a natural component of the human condition and nurses are called to be as a result of that suffering. Many times over, human suffering will present itself; it is the nature of this path. Once your own comfort level resolves itself, it will enable you to encounter greater suffering with the opportunity to observe greater healing within others and within your own self.

I have seen many people die, but I have also seen many people live. Countless times I have encountered people who come up to me and ask me if I remember them from a time when they were in the hospital and I helped them. Sometimes I remember them and sometimes I don't. To hear people thank me and say that I helped them overcome one of the most difficult experiences of their lives is beyond gratifying. To observe the contrast of someone who occupied death's space and now is vibrating with so much life force is a reward specifically for the one who maintains his/her journey as a servant to others.

Will you choose to participate in this journey? If you have already chosen to begin this journey, will you also choose to stay the course? When it becomes too difficult, will you deviate from it? If you should ever deviate from the Calling, will you choose to return? Many times the Calling will test you in order to refine you and many times you will slip, of that I guarantee. But another guarantee is that there is enough mercy within the graciousness of the Calling to return you to the path that you love, if you so choose to participate. Above all else, our soul seeks to be satiated and I encourage you to seek that which your soul desires. For me, nursing is a part of that spiritual journey and if you are reading this, then "WELCOME" because you have already begun.

Nursing as a Spiritual Practice

It would be necessary for me to introduce how important self-care and self-love is when participating in this experience of nursing. Working in health care is hard and more challenging than most careers. Because nursing has its challenging moments, moments that will try you as a person, moments that will challenge how strong a nurse you really are, it will be vitally necessary for you to have established powerful ways of taking care of yourself.

In those moments when your energy is zapped and your vision is blurred, I hope you will find that quiet place inside of you that has enough wisdom to listen to the song of the Calling. I have personally found that when you sing a song of gratitude right in the middle of chaos, life will respond by fitting you with a new perspective and you can once again enter back into harmony with the Calling. This is how you know if you still love it and how you know it still loves you.

After I had graduated from nursing school, I realized that working in healthcare wasn't just a career for the sake of being a career - it was substantially more than that. I had already been working in the hospital setting for 13 years, and so the nursing environment was not new to me in any capacity. I had just graduated nursing school but was still working as an emergency room technician. One day, as I was entering in and out of patient rooms and encountering various types of personalities, I realized that serving others in this way was not just a thing I did but it was actually becoming a spiritual practice for me. I was entering into people's personal space, discerning what, where and why their pain was present and doing my best to uplift them when I realized in *this* occupation, the art of effectively exchanging and transacting various energies required me to operate out of a very spiritual place.

I began to recognize very consciously that encountering human beings at a time when their physical integrity was being challenged required a more spiritual approach in order to be truly effective. When people are in a weakened state and placed in a strange sterile environment and scrutinized by strangers, all the while enduring physical pain, a storm of emotions can rise to the surface, especially fear. Fear can manifest as impatience, anger, sorrow, tears, stoicism, or even violence. If one is not operating out of a true "soul space" then after awhile, it becomes humanly impossible for the healthcare practitioner to authentically encounter each person with the appropriate amount of respect and physical/emotional support it takes to be a stellar caretaker. Nursing floors especially are breeding grounds for stress, because a tremendous amount of quality work that is physical, emotional and intellectual in nature needs to be done constantly the *entire* shift. Not only must you encounter the patient's fluctuating physical and emotional circumstances. But you are also interacting with many coworkers and team members who all contribute a diverse energy to the environment. As it is necessary for nurses to be team players, we have accountability to our co-workers as well, a responsibility to see the wealth of spirit and intelligence they have to offer our patients and us. Yet, in times when the workload is overwhelming, undesired personality traits can manifest and alter the energetic tone of a previously balanced work environment.

When the balance of the environment shifts and your self-control is at its limit, you will need to quickly access a place of greater resource to maintain the floor *and* your sanity. Nursing can rapidly become something that annoys you if you aren't fully aware of *why* you're a nurse and what the practice of nursing actually means to you. Nursing is a spiritual practice for *me* and I am passionate about protecting it with tremendous love and care.

Nursing *is* my spiritual practice. In my choosing to participate and respond to the Call, there is a deep joy that is generated as a result. Not a joy that makes you jump up and down, but I mean a sort of joy that goes deeper, a sense of satisfaction that I am doing what I am supposed to do at the exact season in my life that I am supposed to be doing it. In the authentic approach to nursing, there is a positive feedback loop that is created and must be maintained by self-care, self-love and selflessness in order to produce a quality nurse. Truly, what I give to my practice returns gracefully and harmoniously back into me, and therein is how my mind, body and spirit are sustained for the work at hand.

For every well-rounded person, it would be said that there is an established balance between his or her body, mind and spirit. Before one can become a truly balanced healer, one must first discover a balance in his/her beingness. It is true that the grandeur of every great thing is laid up in the tiny details. It is the investment to each and every stroke that can produce a work such as a Mona Lisa. As a nurse, in order for you to move in harmony you need to also invest in the tiny details that connect the body, mind and spirit. Out of these three pillars that support the consciousness, it is the mind that is the most difficult to care for.

The mind is a powerful and complex environment. Depending on how you interact with your mind will determine how you show up in the world. On one hand, the mind is simply the central nervous system made up of billions of neurons electronically communicating with each other for the means of survival. Essentially, that *is* what it is on a cellular level, but it is so much more than that. The mind is an organic computer storing all of your experiences as "memory." It is the temple for the egoic part of us. The mind can be the vehicle that parks you in the position of being a nurse, but it is not the sole contributor. We need the mind to store facts within itself as "our memory" in order for the scientist parts of being a healthcare worker to be present, but curiously enough it is equally important to know how to step away from the mind in order to be effective.

Part of caring for one's mind is knowing how to quiet, abandon, or resolve the intense interaction that can come with warring thoughts. It is within the field of "mind" that self-doubt, pride, hurt, fear, anxiety, aggression and opinionated mindsets take root. How is it possible to utilize the same tool to build and also breakdown? Curious and fascinating. People have found ways of creating peaceful mindsets to navigate around this, meditation and prayer being among the healthier ways.

Having been in healthcare for 14 years, and currently working as an emergency room nurse, I have seen some of the unhealthiest ways and their unfortunate outcomes of those attempting to escape an imbalanced mind. Drugs, alcohol, sex, suppression of thoughts and aggression towards others can numb the mind but cannot cultivate balance or environments for quality growth. Unnecessary mind clutter is usually a result of faulty relationship dynamics with family, friends, partners, co-workers, money and with oneself. Typically, our unresolved issues release their negative energy when one's environment is stressful, as during these times, we lose the ability to keep what is unresolved in our lives hidden, thus the energetic toxicity of our issues is released into the energetic field of our work environment. In my own experience, I have found that slipping into the awareness that I am the "observer of the thoughts," and not the "actual thoughts," that offers quick relief. When I operate in the knowingness that I am the "observer of the experience," and not stake my claim or identity as the "result of that experience," that I am offered an escape from how loud the mind can be. With continual practice this will result in a more peaceful and balanced way of interacting with ones own mind and with others.

When the job at hand requires you to be fully present; for example, like during a code or a very busy shift, you need to be able to push away warring and distracting thoughts in order to be fully effective. By operating as the "soul awareness," instead of the egoic mind, you can access what you need from memory without splitting your attention between what is important and what is unnecessary mind clutter.

Those that continually work at establishing a healthy relationship with their mind can extend that effort to a quality relationship with the body. It is no secret that working in healthcare has tremendous effects on the physical body. The work some days can be physically laborious and the hours doing these tasks can be for many hours, if not the entire shift. I have seen nurses allow their bodies to go from young and strong to overweight and weak. I have seen nurses over the years go from able-bodied to barely being able to shuffle in for shift, back bent and cane in hand. In conjunction, exercising, stretching and strengthening techniques to keep the body limber need to be established for longevity when working at the bedside. I encourage you to listen to your body as it has so much to tell you. The relationship between you and your body is just as important as the relationship between you and your mind. One exposes the love of being a nurse by taking care of the body of the nurse. The body is a temple for the soul, and food that is worthy fuel needs to be consumed if the body is to carry out the complete work that life has lovingly called you to do.

It is, of course, your spirit that produces the intensity at which your body and mind will engage all of the opportunities presented to you. It is because of this that a quality spiritual discipline is beneficial. Some choose a religion or meditative practice, but what ever it is that you choose in order to feed your spiritual force, it must be nutritious in order to produce growth. Too religious and your egoic mind will parade as a false sense of spirituality. Too inclined to meditation and you will want to avoid interaction with others. It is your responsibility to find the appropriate balance in spiritual discipline in order to be energetically palatable to your patients and your coworkers. If you are unsure on how to encourage and build your internal spirit I recommend starting at a place of acute silence and listening.

In reality, our soul craves the silence of its own beautiful self. We know this because there is an intense satisfaction with falling into deep sleep. Within deep sleep, we abandon our mind, we leave behind our body and enter into a quiet place, and when we awaken, we are refreshed. When the soul spends time within the silence of itself, it is recharged. When we know how to be ourselves, minus our convoluted mindsets, perceptions and judgments, we present with a *cleaner* energy that our patients can feel safe enough in while exposing their vulnerabilities. When our soul knows the peace of its own presence, when the sea of our mind is stilled and when our body is healthy, a true healer can appear in the nurse, *as* the nurse.

When the egoic-mind is put aside and allows the "soul space" to take the reins of our lives, we become a force that now has true power to create healing environments. Out of this space comes the selfless love that it takes to be a true nurse. It is the soul that knows how to harmonize with all forces and situations it encounters. When nurses ride the waves of their own Calling, in this particular light, they can step into any situation and bring it into a more balanced state.

I have found that the soul has an interesting way of connecting us to those in need. It would be nice to say that we enter into each patient's life as a shining beacon of light representing spiritual, physical and mental health. The reality is that we must bring everything that humbles us as we enter into their lives. It is this beautiful weight that connects our humanity to the patient's humanity, as we are no greater or better than anyone lying in a hospital bed. Our bodies are subject to disease, just as theirs are. Yet, if we achieve within our own self a greater balance in body, mind and spirit, then our weights can be weightless and operate as an incredible benefit to our practice. The truth is that we are also human and therefore exposed to experiences that can cause pain. Pain can be a thing that refines our own personal seeing, which allows us to identify that struggle in others and create a safe space for another to expose and heal in. If we allow gratitude to enter into our lives for our struggle, then we can transcend our pain and carry with us the satisfaction of being one that overcomes. It is with this sense of empowered humility that allows the component of leadership within the healer to beckon the one who is in a state of peril towards the path of health. One who is balanced and present can assist in bringing balance to another's mind or spirit even before relief is brought to their body.

One excellent way that a good healthcare worker can establish balance in suffering patients and their family members is by allowing humor to be infused within their practice. Humor insights laughter, and when done out of good intention, can produce a bridge between a healthcare worker and the patient. The powerful thing about laughter is that while it's happening, it causes the mind to be silenced. Thoughts of worry cannot race through when someone is enjoying laughter. I encourage everyone to laugh as much as they can. I always say if I don't have at least one good belly laugh during my day, I wasn't doing it right. Of course I am not saying to go and make your abdominal surgery patient go into a fit of belly laughs (insert side eye), but what I'm saying is that you have an opportunity to show the patient that you care about their mental and spiritual disposition while they are under your care. Not only does this build a therapeutic relationship between you and your patient, but it also gives your own mind and spirit a great opportunity to enjoy and relish the human interaction that comes with being a nurse. This unique type of interaction is also a pertinent part of caring for your own self, as funny as that sounds. You have to enjoy the work!

One thing that I have learned about working in the emergency room is that it will require (and I repeat, REQUIRE) you to have a sense of humor. I don't mean a sense of cynicism, or "dark" humor, but I mean a healthy and robust way of living and seeing, even when the dark spaces encroach themselves upon our lives. A healthy sense of humor will never laugh *at* someone but, rather, *with* someone. For example, just the other day I was working with a diabetic patient whose right arm had been amputated a number of years earlier. During his stay, he and I had a number of lighthearted conversations and I was glad when he became open to the education I gave him on how to manage his diabetes. As I was taking out the IV in his left hand, he tells me, "You have no idea how many times a nurse has asked to me to hold down the gauze with my right hand. I mean, really?" I discerned that this man was not actually upset about it and really just thought it was kind of silly. Within moments, he, his family, and myself were cracking up a storm like old friends. There will not always be opportunities to laugh in such awkward situations, but when the opportunities present themselves, jump in fully! In that moment, he knew he could trust me with his vulnerability because of the way that I energetically encountered him during his stay. It is *THIS* type of interaction that we nurses live for!

Nursing is *my* spiritual practice. It is within this spiritual practice that the art of human interaction arises. Professionalism arises in this spiritual practice. The healer arises in this spiritual practice. The scientist arises in this spiritual practice. Joy, sorrow, laughter, tears and the mosaic of the human experience arises in *this* practice. As I said before, in my *choosing* to participate and respond to the Call, there is a joy that is generated as a result. In the authentic approach to nursing, there is a positive feedback loop that is created, a feedback loop that my soul takes responsibility for. I choose to take accountability for my nursing practice by covering and tending to it with care and love in order for it to operate at optimal function. For all of the hard work that I have poured out of myself in order to have this honor, I am blessed one-thousand times over. The ultimate gift that life gives the nurse is that in the participation of doing what we love, we have the strong sense of coming home.

About The Author

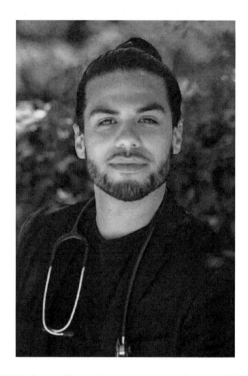

Emilio Vigil, RN is a Bay Area native from California. He has worked in health care for fourteen years and currently works as an emergency room nurse. Emilio is passionate about encouraging those who hear the Calling to be a nurse to purse that dream. He believes with hard work, dedication and a good sense of humor, anything can be accomplished.

To Contact the Author:

Mr.Emilio.Vigil@gmail.com

CHAPTER 7

From CNA to Entrepreneur

My name is Itaska Shoffner and this is what made me want to work in the healthcare field to become a CNA.

It all started in 1999 when my mother had a heart attack and had to have open-heart surgery. At the time, I had relocated to Indianapolis, IN. I received a call from my grandmother, telling me that my mother had to be rushed to the hospital and that she would update me on things. I asked her if I needed to come back and she said no, not yet but she would let me know. My grandmother called me later that evening updating me on my mother's progress. She said that my mother had to have emergency surgery because she had a heart attack.

Once she was ready to be up in her wheelchair per doctor's orders, she was. While she was up in her wheelchair, something fell, so she pushed her call light and waited but no one answered. So she tried to pick it up herself and fell out of her wheelchair and still no one ever answered her call light. My mother started to call out, "HELP ME" because she was bleeding from her surgery site. She could not pull herself up because she was too weak, so she lay there until someone came to check on her, but still no one answered her call light during this process. Where was family during all this, right? My grandmother had to leave to check on my son and nephew and she was in need of a break. Someone did make it into her room and asked why she did not call out. My mother said that she did but no one ever answered and the famous response was that they were sorry and everyone was busy. The nurse rushed to go call the doctor and he came up to my mother's room. She had busted open a few stitches from her falling and the doctor stated that he was going to stitch her back up. My mother was unaware that it was going to happen right in the room and asked the doctor if he needed to make sure things were sterile. The doctor stated that she was going to be fine but she was not so sure and didn't like his answer. After the doctor was finished, she called my grandmother and told her what had just happened to her and that she was scared to be left there alone.

My grandmother went back to the hospital and asked to speak with the person in charge and that she wanted to speak with the doctor, also. She talked with the person in charge, who was very apologetic about no one coming in to assist my mother and what they would do the next time to prevent a fall. My grandmother was so mad and didn't like her answer and said some choice words and demanded to speak with the doctor, but was told he was busy in surgery. After that, he was busy every time grandmother or myself would try to contact him and we could only speak with his nurse. My grandmother never left my mother's bedside after that and watched everything that was being done or not done.

When the time came for my mother to be discharged home, we were so happy because she was not happy with her care there. She was doing fine the first week she was home. The next week, my mother started to not feel well and caught a temperature. My grandmother called me and let me know what was going on with my mother. I said if she still had a temperature in a few days to call the doctor, and she said okay. And a few days later, she still had the temperature and she had started to smell a foul odor and she was having drainage coming from the incision. I asked her a few questions about how she looked and how often was she having to change her dressing. She stated that a spot had opened up and it was getting larger and she had to pack it very often. I said I was going to call her back because I was going to call the doctor. Long story short, they said that once they had contacted the doctor and given orders on what to do, they were going to call us back. I hung up that phone to head back to Gary, knowing that they were going to do nothing, and I felt like she would die being under their care any longer. I know Gary is two hours from Indianapolis, but I'm sure I got there in about an hour.

When I got to Gary, my mother's eyes looked as if they had sunk into her head and she looked as if she was dying. I called that doctor back and no, I was not nice about what I had to say. The nurse told us to bring her back and they would be waiting for her. I hung up yet again and called my aunt in Indianapolis and asked for the name of the doctor that had cared for my mother years back when she had her first heart attack in 1993. I explained to my aunt how my mother looked and that I was scared to take her back to the hospital in Gary. She told me that she would call me back and that it was going to be okay. I waited for what seemed to be a long time; actually, it wasn't, but to me, it felt as if it took years to hear back. As the phone was ringing, I could hear an ambulance. I answered and it was my aunt and the doctor on the phone. I explained what was going on and what my mother was looking like. The doctor was telling me that an ambulance was on the way and that it would get to Indianapolis as soon as possible. I said to her the ambulance sounded like they were outside and

Chapter 7

she said that they would be waiting and that she would see me soon. When I got off the phone, all I could do was cry because I felt I was not there for my mother because I had to work. We followed the ambulance back to Indianapolis and there was a team of doctors, nurses and respiratory, waiting for us. All I know is that everyone was running so fast that I felt I could not keep up. Once we got to a door, a nurse stopped and said that she was going to take me to another room where I could wait until they were done. I remembered her giving me a big hug and saying that she was going to stay with me until they were done. I so appreciated that but unbeknownst to me, my family was there, waiting as well. We waited what seemed like a century. When the doctors did come out, they let everyone know that she was stable and had we made it a minute later she would not have lived. They also stated that they could not perform the surgery due to what was already done. They had to contact a team of doctors out of the country to perform the surgery they could not do. It took some weeks or longer for the team of doctors to make it to the States. They kept my family informed every step of the way. I was by mother's bedside day in and day out this time around. I sat there and just talked to her, even though she could not respond. When the doctor came to inform me that the team had made it to the States and would be performing the surgery in a few days, I was scared and happy at the same time.

We are a praying family and we believed and had faith that she would recover from this. After surgery, she was placed on a ventilator and had chest tubes in. I continued to talk with her about any and everything. I thought back to how things took place at the other hospital and how unhappy I was with how she was treated. I shared with my mother that I wanted to help people who couldn't take care of themselves. I had this Thrifty Nickel paper and saw a class to take to become a CNA. I said to my mother that that was what I wanted to do and that I was going to look into it. So, as time went on and they removed my mother from the ventilator and the chest tubes, I was excited because I could not wait to hear my mother's voice and look into her eyes. I knew that she had a long journey ahead of her and that I was along for the ride. The doctor said she would have about 6 months of rehab and that it might get hard but to keep fighting. The care my mother received was amazing and I was comfortable leaving her when I had something to do, even though there was family there every day. My mother was a fighter, so I knew she was not going to let it keep her down. Once she was transferred to a nursing home for her rehab, my family and I came up with who would take what shift. I signed up for the CNA class and I could not wait to tell her, because she was all for it.

It was hard going to the classes, being a mother and caring for my mother, but I made it happen. I noticed how some did not have the heart or compassion to be in the health care field. I would say to my mother I would never treat people like they were treating some of the residents. The CNAs lacked knowledge and some of the nurses were just above doing bedside care. I would talk with some of the CNAs to find out what made them want to get into the healthcare field and what were the challenges they faced. As for the challenges, a lot would respond short staffing, or they felt that they were unappreciated by the nurses and that management didn't care. I took a mental note of things, not to be on the fence, but to know how to prepare myself. Once my

Chapter 7

mother was released home, she had homecare set up for her and I wanted to know everything I needed to know to care for her. Caring for my mother made me even more excited to become a CNA. As the time went on and I finished the class and became certified, I was ready to work.

I applied at a nursing home and they called me back so fast that I was, like, okay yes, I'm ready, but then I was thinking about the short staff issue I was warned about. I still was ready and knew I would give it my all. I also knew I couldn't change things but I wanted to make some kind of difference. Working in long-term care was hard and it could take a toll on you, your heart and body. I was the one who went in smiling, speaking to everyone and wanting to help. It didn't take me long to catch on to things and see how they took my kindness for weakness. There were so many days I went into work and wanted to walk back out. My heart would break because a lot of the residents didn't have family who came to visit and some did. There were many days when we didn't have the supplies needed to perform good continuity of care. One day, I was so not feeling it, and when I got my report, my assignment was a mess. I went to talk with the administrator, because I had voiced my concerns to the DON and it went over her head. I asked him how he expected CNAs to do their job when they didn't have what was needed. I also stated that the teamwork was just not there at all; the nurses were above us and their job was to only pass meds and do treatments. I was so frustrated talking to him that I'm sure my words came off wrong, but I had had it. I also stated that I felt, as a new or old CAN, we needed to have ongoing training and education in case of a code. I told him I didn't feel comfortable performing CPR because when you don't use it, you lose it. He had a look, like, who do you think you are, walking into my office and telling me what needs to be done in my facility? After our talk, I felt better because at least he knew where I was coming from even if the others were scared to voice their opinion.

After that, I knew I wanted to do more and learn more because I was just not okay with where I was. I continued to work in long-term care for about 2 ½ years before I started applying at hospitals. While working in hospitals, I gained as much experience as I could. I worked in hospitals for 16 ½ years before I was actually ready to step out on faith and pursue my dreams of being an entrepreneur. Many thoughts ran through my head about what kind of business and where to start. I knew I wanted to do something in the healthcare field, but just didn't know where to start. I started researching the transportation field and I saw that there was a need for it in my area. During my research, my mother became ill again and I put what I wanted to do on hold because I had to take time off from my job so that I could care for her, which was very important to me. It wasn't much longer after I took the time off that she was declining and I was not ready for this. She was a fighter so I thought that she was going to be ok and fight through this. My mother had overcome many bumps and never let anything keep her down - not even her disability.

One day I couldn't wake her up and I thought it was just her blood sugar after I took it and it didn't register. I called 911 while still trying to arouse her. I took her blood pressure and I couldn't hear anything because it was faint. The ambulance came and rushed her to the hospital where they got her stable. She was

Chapter 7

admitted and stayed for about two weeks. The level of care she received was awful - they expected her to feed herself! And I just couldn't wrap my head around how you would expect someone in my mother's condition to feed herself. One nurse stated to me that they knew I was there and that is why they didn't feed her. I told her and her tray was delivered at 5:30 pm. Now it was 7 pm…why did she have to wait, anyway, even if I was there? There were a number of things taking place that were neglectful. To see so much of what is happening in healthcare just made me sad, because we put our loved ones in the hands of professionals and expect for them to be treated fairly and with dignity. I had her transferred to another hospital and I felt a lot better. I just wanted her to be taken care of; that wasn't asking for much because it was their job.

Once released home, she needed to be rushed back out and I knew then something else going on. Things took a turn for the worst and she was back on the ventilator. After a couple of days, they removed her but then she had to go back on after they coded her about 4 times, I think. The hardest choice was removing her from the ventilator after being told she wouldn't recover. Being on the other side was so hard because I was able to see first hand what other families went through. The staff was great and went above and beyond to care for my mother and assist our family.

After she passed, it hit me hard and my focus wasn't on my journey of entrepreneurship. It took me a little over a year to get back on my journey and to shift my mindset. Four years later, I knew what it was I wanted to do. I saw the need for seniors and disabled people who want to age in their own homes. I researched that market and felt that I would love to get into that business - to help those in need. I went through the whole process of researching and attending a class to teach me the laws for my state and how to write my policies and procedures and just to learn how to start and run the business. The non-medical homecare business is very much needed, but it's a very saturated market. I had to figure out what was my niche and what would set me apart from all the others. What was I going to bring that was different? I feel strongly that if God called me to it, then there's room for me.

I thought about things and knew that I didn't want to stay in Indianapolis after my son graduated. So I put my plan for my homecare business on hold. Shortly thereafter, my grandmother passed away. One day I was talking with my cousin and sharing with her that in order for me to be able to start up my homecare company, I needed the funds to support it. She shared with me that I should look into the uniform business and it would help fund my homecare business. So I did and I made the decision that this was a great idea and it was of great demand in the healthcare industry. I did my research for this business and did everything to make my business legal. There were a few bumps in the road but I refused to give up. I continued to surround myself with likeminded people who inspired me to be better. I am determined to grow my business and give it my all. I am excited to introduce "Uniquely Scrubs" to the world!

Self-care & Self-Love

Self-care & Self-love: What that means for me and what I did to change some things in my life.

When it comes to taking care of myself, I have always put myself last, which is very easy to do when you're used to being the caregiver for everyone else. Self-care is very important because we need to take care of ourselves in order to keep going in life, yet it is something about which people forget. I would be so focused on others and so worn out that I would be, like, forget about me for now - I'll get to me on this day or that day…and that day never came. I now know that what I needed was balance, which I didn't know how to add in my life at the time. So, with the stress of life and day-to-day activities of being a single mother, it was tough on me. I was happy, yet unhappy at times and I just could not figure out why and what was going on with me. I knew that if I let go of a toxic relationship, that would lift me up out of a situation from which I needed to be free so I could love me. One day, I said to myself, look now - it's time for a sit down and evaluate what's happening in your life. I was very deserving and worthy of putting myself first, but I did not know how to do so and tell others "no." I took steps that were small but they were huge for me! I started saying "no" and once I did, things slowed down in my life. I was able to have room for my thoughts and me and I started to focus on my health, my goals and my dreams and that alone made me feel productive. My stress level went down because I was not running around for people, all crazy, and I wasn't sick from colds or tired all time. I did not realize that just by taking time out of my day made a big difference. I just completely removed things and people that caused me more stress. I had to learn what things I liked, enjoyed and the happiness and peace within myself.

I noticed that my skin started to clear up and my hair was on the right track of growing very healthy. I gained weight but I was fine with my size - it was my stomach area but then my doctor stated to me that stress and drinking soda pop could cause my weight gain in that area. As time passed, I noticed that I had started slimming down. I am not a person that diets, but what I did do was watch how much food I ate at a time and drink more water. People around me noticed the glow I had and how I looked in the clothes I wore and yes, that put a smile on my face and made me happy for my new changes. I have poor sleep habits so I would read and drink a hot cup of tea before going to bed to help me relax. I'm a thinker and my mind is always wondering about life, even when I'm sleeping, so I would be exhausted in the mornings. Me getting proper rest at night helped me feel better during the day. I would write down ways and things to help me be a better person than I was yesterday and apply it in my life. I had to learn to stop making excuses for things not going right in my life and I started making things happen. My friends would invite me out and I would make every excuse in the world not to go because I was used to just staying in the house. I never paid any mind to how important it was to get out and socialize. I did not know that I was isolating myself from others by declining invites, but because it was normal for me, I didn't think twice about it. Well, it's not good to do that because it is also a form of depression and loneliness and could lead to other things. I have learned to talk about things and not keep them bottled up inside of me. I take myself out on a "me date." At first it was strange, but after a few times, I noticed others did the same thing. I write my thoughts down, to free my mind, and I read as well, so to buy books is something that I really enjoy. I take long baths just to relax my mind and have alone time. I love lighting candles, so it's normal for me and something I do coming in the door once I am off work, because it just makes me feel at peace in my home. I cry sometimes, and not because I'm sad but because it's good to do that from time to time. I have a favorite song by Mary J Blige, *Just Fine*. When I tell you that song makes me feel good and want to get up and dance or something, it is an understatement. I will play that song when I'm in my car and turn it all the way up. I pray on a daily basis, and without God and prayer, I wouldn't have made it through some of the storms I did. I just know that if I'm not healthy and in good condition, I can't be around for my son and nephew when they need me. The things I do for me work for me and make me happy and I will continue to do what makes me feel good inside and out. Anything that's negative does not have a welcome card in my life, so I do not give my good energy to certain things. The more I take care of my body, the more it will reward me in the end.

I also feel that self-care and self-love shouldn't feel like work, but just a way of life. To invest in yourself first does not have to be lavish and expensive, but sometimes if that's what you want, you deserve it, so why not? So, as long as I keep balance and I rejuvenate myself, I can take on anything. Putting you first and doing what makes you happy inside and out is what matters. Our health is top priority and we have to pay attention to it even when we feel we don't have the time or money. Due to going through some difficult times in my life, I had to rebuild myself into the strong woman that I am today. I will never allow myself to go back and deal with certain things, but I will say it made me stronger. I love me, inside and out, and I don't need validation from anyone about that. See, there was a time in my life when I didn't feel this way. I had lost my confidence but people never knew because I didn't show that side of me. I say this to say love you, no matter who doesn't.

About the Author

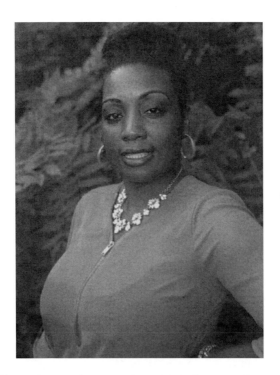

Itaska Shoffner (born August 29, 1980) is a native of Gary, IN. She is a mother of two - son Malcolm L. Mitchell, Jr. and nephew Ja'Quan M. Shoffner. Itaska is a CNA and entrepreneur. She began her journey in healthcare as a CNA in January of 2000. She enjoyed caring for others wherever there was a need. Aside from being a caregiver, she always knew there was more she wanted to do with her life. Years later, she took the leap of faith and pursued her dreams of becoming an entrepreneur, and that's where Uniquely Scrubs was formed in 2018. Itaska currently resides in Indianapolis, IN.

To contact The Author:

ItaskaShoffner@yahoo.com

www.uniquelyscrubs.shop

uniquelyscrubsllc@gmail.com

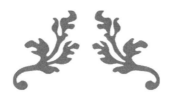

CHAPTER 8

Lil' Lisa

Imagine the ending of a hot, humid summer in the late 60's, when most teenagers are eager to go back to school. Well, this particular one was preparing to give birth. An unwed, uneducated 16 year old, living in the deep South. There is nothing really abnormal about this except for me, the little girl born into this dysfunctional formation called a family.

The date was September 26, 1967 and the nearest medical facility to handle women ready to give birth was in the next county. My birth mother gave me a name no one could pronounce; as I later found out, she (the birth mother) was trying to copy or emulate a distant cousin's name. Her name was Melissa. Sooo, being the quirky teenager that she was, she decided to put a twist on it and replace the "M" with an "F"…hmmm. As the white nurses in the rural southern hospital condescendingly questioned the exhausted, impoverished 16 year old about the spelling, pronunciation, etc., she mumbled something that was recorded as "Flessie," but at some point became "Felissia," pronounced "Felicia"…and so it begins.

The family quickly shortened that nonsensical blurb to what I have been known to answer to for the last 50 years - Lisa.

That introduction is the foundation for a life that was conceived out of immaturity, hatred and jealousy. AJ (my mother) was the 15 year old, middle child of 6, jockeying for a position in typical middle-child syndrome and feeling excluded. Being a straight A student at school did not even register a raised eyebrow or a "congratulations," not from her father, as this was expected. Mr.

Chapter 8

Dave was a big man and carried a pistol. He often times cashed checks, back when people of color did not have banking credentials, so he cashed their checks for them as he often carried large amounts of cash. He sired 6 children by Carolyn and was rumored to have had more. He was the true definition of a rolling stone. Daddy Dave only dropped by occasionally to spend the night and/or to dish out discipline. This interaction between her parents set in motion a lifelong craving for attention and acceptance. AJ was academically smarter than her siblings and was easily bored with school. She often set out to walk to town, which was barely a county mile away on the dirt road. AJ had seen this older, handsome, well-dressed boy looking at her on more than one occasion. This particular day, it was sweltering hot and AJ was enjoying an ice cream cone. Ray saw her and quickly began to purse her. Five to six months of courtship ensued and by May of 1967, shortly before her 16th birthday, AJ was pregnant.

Ray's parents were educated professionals and AJ was not quite what they had envisioned. The two families lived only a mere 5 miles apart and were separated by a railroad track. I made my entrance to a loving and caring set of paternal grandparents. They accepted me from day one and took me and raised me to be what I am today. Values and morals that escaped the teenager were instilled in me by the very people AJ despised. She wanted to use me as a pawn to extort some of life's finer things from the well-to-do family. My toy box was running over and there was not a shortage of love. AJ's plan had somewhat backfired and she was no match for the seasoned hard-core parents that wanted to make the best out of an already awkward situation. There was not a lot of resistance, as AJ was now able to complete school and hang out with her friends, as if nothing had happened. She was having so much fun she got pregnant again 3 years later by someone else, and again 3 years after that (with twins) by someone else.

Lil' Lisa navigated through this fairly well, without a lot of residual baggage. She is currently pursing entrepreneurial and professional dreams and uses the backdrop of her childhood as a kaleidoscope for future murals of testimony for a life worth living, regardless how it started.

About The Author

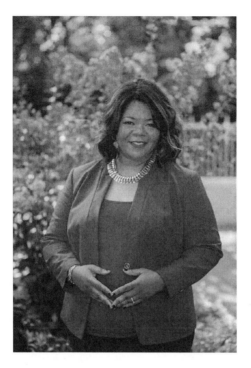

Felissia Felder is a licensed vocational nurse who also holds a bachelor's degree in Healthcare Administration. Throughout her 17 year nursing career, Felissia has worked in orthopedics, medical-surgical, long-term care and is currently working in case management. Felissia has recently attained a certificate of training for HEDIS and the National Gerontology certification. When Felissia is not catching up on a good read, she loves to travel and cook with her husband and kids.

To Contact the Author:

ffelder95@gmail.com
Felderconsultantfrim.com

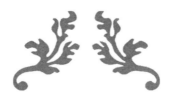

CHAPTER 9

Poised on Purpose

Hopscotch, hide and seek, double-dutch, spin the bottle…all the games of my childhood. There was nothing like hearing my friends banging down my screen door in the morning asking, "Can you come out and play?" I wanted to be a part of the crowd - included, considered good enough, cool, down, not the weird one and, did I say, liked?

Looking back over the chapters of my life, I've discovered, 50+ years later, the game never really changes. Not just the game, but also the desire and the need to belong, to be a part of what is believed to be the "right" crowd. These feelings and emotions would prove to be my tour guide, the hostess with the most-est, influencing many of the decisions I'd make shaping my experiences, my relationships and illuminating what some would call today, my "brand," but what is also known as good old reputation.

College was a major decision. Not if I was going - there was never a doubt I was going to college. I still don't know what other options would have existed for me because my parents never allowed my brain to think of anything else. It was automatic in my house that after high school came college. I chose what seemed to be an obvious school, but it was really the first adult version of hide and go seek in which I would choose to engage. My decision was laced in the need to find something that I could no longer find. I chose to chase the comfort of well-known relationships and rejection, and search for the comfort of familiarity and low risk. I will never forget the excitement and nervousness that college brought. There were new and very different people, a higher level of partying, cramming and freedom. As a freshman in college, my suspicions were confirmed - it's all about what you know, who you know and what you do with that information.

Amidst all the game playing in college, I played some and some were played on me. I was able to come up for air and make a few decisions that set my career journey onto a great path. I honed in on the upper classmen who appeared to have it going on. I listened to how people on campus spoke of them, how they set themselves apart from the norm. I realized they had their game together and I secretly followed their paths. I decided to take a semester away from school, move to a new town where I really knew no one and participate in an internship program. Still wanting to graduate "on-time," I also committed to summer school to make up the hours and classes I would enjoy missing. At that time, the best way to secure a job in time for graduation was having relevant work experience. My focus at that time was short-term: to secure a job before I graduated, not realizing that I had just set myself up for long-term success. I wasn't cognizant of it at the time but I was demonstrating a level of independence and risk taking. The internship paid off, yielding a job offer from every company with whom I interviewed. The idea of Los Angeles, California excited me most. By the time I received that job offer, I had made another major life decision: to get married at the age of 22. I held onto the decision to get married and let go of the opportunity to move to California. I still have those "coulda, woulda, shoulda" thoughts about the decision. I turned down the West Coast for the Midwest and my desire to be married forever.

Working in downtown Chicago and living on the north side in a high rise on the lake was a young professional's marvel. I didn't think much of California at that time, not even on those harsh winter mornings on the express bus looking at the frozen lake. There's just something about the city of Chicago that you can't find in other major cities. I worked for a major retailer in their flagship store. I met a number of people, including Oprah Winfrey and Michael Jordan, who were, themselves, newcomers to Chicago at the time. The exposure was more than I ever expected and the life lessons, both professionally and personally, started to take shape as well. I realized I had a gift of discernment, understanding those with whom you need to connect professionally and those from whom you need to run. I formed informal mentoring relationships with key leaders in business but also with seasoned front line staff. It was that group, the well seasoned, who really kept their hands on the pulse of what was happening in business and held their deep historical perspective filed away for someone willing to listen, like me. They always wanted to help the new kid, wanted to "teach" you what you really needed to know and what they weren't going to teach me in that development program I was in. I remained open to all their wisdom and discarded what wasn't for me while holding on to the nugget that would take me where I really wanted to play. I maintained those relationships and sat at their feet for every drop of information they were willing to share.

Professionally, I was learning, gaining exposure and feeling good about the future, and yet, personally, I was struggling. There was so much newness and at the same time I found myself re-playing this same game of Double Dutch. By this time, I had matured enough to know, or maybe I was just tired of the game, but I gained an inkling that it was more important that I love myself; at least that's what all the magazines were telling me. There had come a time in this very moment when it was time to care more about myself, rather than the feeling of belonging just to belong. I needed to remove the chip from my brain that had me consumed with the idea of needing to prove something to people who really didn't matter and to people who didn't like me for their own twisted reasons. I had to stop living the double life, the one I allowed my family to see and the real one I tried to keep hidden. Plus, I've never been that good at jumping Double Dutch. Standing firmly on my own two feet always proved best for me, so I walked away from my marriage with 2 beautiful babies in my arms, a budding career and a head and heart of fear and confusion. I could say a lot of things in my head, but honestly, the heart was a different matter altogether.

Divorce was not an easy decision; hiding the reasons for the divorce from co-workers and family was extremely difficult. I had two people in my life that I could share everything with - my earthly lifelines. Those special individuals who allowed me to decompress, who challenged me, had my back and told me when I was coming off the track. This decision forced me to develop double vision. I needed vision for my new family structure, for these two lives I pledged to care for. I needed to be a good example to them, a role model, a steady. I also had to gain vision from a professional perspective. I mean, we had to eat so I had to maintain my career. Now that I was a single mother, a barrage of questions started to role through my head, like I was in the middle of Times Square. Would I be limited in what I could do in my career? If I focused on my career would I lose my kids? What opportunities would I be able to take advantage of? Can I balance all of this? What do I need to avoid? Can I be in a relationship? Will my parents approve? Do I care? Should I care? There was a constant tension between my career choices and being engaged as a parent. I'll admit, I didn't chaperone or help out enough at school activities. The balancing act was stressful, and, at times, frustrating. Through all of the haze and the questions, I kept my two lifelines close by at all times and I created The Village. This is the group of individuals who would surround my two heartbeats and me and fill in the gap. Yet, above all that I thought I was doing to prepare and manage, I know that I was protected, guided and shielded by the Almighty during those difficult days.

A change in marital status; why not a change in jobs, too? I found myself running from myself and finding myself, all at the same time. I never considered myself a scrappy type of girl, but big change, hurt and desperation will bring a lot out of you. Through a few emotional bumps and bruises and self-doubt, I discovered I was a survivor. I had a supportive family, The Village, but I also had something to prove. I had to show them when they came knocking on my screen door this time, asking if I could come out and play, that I had my game face on, positioned to show everyone knocking that I had not missed a beat. Underneath it all, I was still consumed with being liked, accepted and part of the end crowd.

My focus was on double vision - my kids and my career. I pursued career opportunities and different organizations. I accepted assignments that placed me on the road multiple days a week, and because of my supportive village, I never had to say "no." Holding on to what I learned earlier in my career, I immediately secured mentors, internal and external to the organization, and both personal and professional. I was clear, within the first 9-12 months, what role within the organization I wanted next. I prepared for it and fostered relationships along the way.

Being consistent, hard working and result oriented all proved to be instrumental in shaping my corporate brand. From department to department, organization to organization and person to person, I heard people using the same words to describe me, my work and my character - fair, honest, get it done. As I advanced in my career, I also intentionally took steps back to expand my knowledge and set me on a new trajectory of growth.

These attributes became my core and began to align my behaviors, reactions and responses, in both my professional and personal life. The lines that I had worked so hard to create, professionally and personally, were blurred. By allowing this crosspollination, I witnessed the impact on my teenagers, how they made decisions, what was important to them, and most importantly, how they treated other people. They were demonstrating a strong sense of discernment and judgment, in many areas. Although I had intentionally acquired this double vision approach as a security net, I soon came to the realization that you become what you focus on. What you focus your attention on will have a direct impact on every aspect of your life.

Like in any game, there are rules if you want to have any chance of coming out on the winning side. You need to have your strategy.

My strategy was, and continues to be, staying surrounded by people who genuinely love and care about me, honoring my word, making mistakes - as long as I learned from each one - and remaining grounded in my relationship with God. It's clear to me now that woven throughout the intricacies of each decision I make are what I now call the pearls of my purpose.

My Perfect Peace

This is what I strive for each day. "I just want a little peace and quiet" is what I grew up hearing, and I found myself saying it as well - over and over again. I don't know what I expected someone else to do about my needs. Did they even understand what peace actually meant to me? I doubt it because my definition of peace continues to change as I change. I had to start by discovering what really brought me joy. Not happiness, but joy. Anyone or anything can take your happiness, but joy, once you get a hold of what that is for you...you will not give that up for anything in the world.

Space and time are my critical paths. Finding the space and time to think, or just be silent, are my must haves. I like road trips. I grew up taking long road trip vacations with my parents - Indiana to California, or Indiana to Mississippi - we took this trip each year on the Fourth of July. This was engrained in me in such a way that I find great comfort in long car rides to this day, as long as the car is moving! Don't get me wrong, I do not like sitting in traffic. One of the most memorable trips for me was a drive from Indiana to Atlanta, GA. I was alone in the car and I started down the interstate thinking about something and never turned the radio on. One hour into the drive I discovered just how much I was enjoying this long moment of silence, the time to really wrestle with my own thoughts and ideas. I turned my cell phone off and continued down the road. I actually found myself totally annoyed when I needed to stop for gas or food. It was a disruption to my creativity. I had to take notes of all the ideas that I was discovering, all dealing with a number of pending tasks and activities colliding in my life at the time. I continued that 10 hour car ride with no music and felt the most refreshed I ever have following that drive. Space and time gives you the permission you need to get into your zone. It is the foundation of anything else you may want to engage in for yourself. It all starts with space and time.

I had to become a blocker to protect my space and time. That means I take control of my time and that also means that I tell some people "NO, not now," or "NO, not ever." In my professional life, that means blocking white space on my calendar and not allowing anyone to schedule over it unless I say it's okay. When I initially tried this, I was nervous, had all kinds of crazy scenarios running around in my head, palms sweating…just crazy talk. When I actually formed my lips to say "no," I heard a voice say "okay, thank you." I couldn't believe it; surely it was not going to be that easy. That moment liberated me; freed me from my secret need to be everything to everyone. I now have a magic word that seems to work miracles, and that word is simply "no."

My joy starts by serving others. There is no deeper spiritual connection than what you experience when serving the needs of others. When I focus on helping, or simply encouraging, I have less time to focus on my stuff. It's a two for one deal. One act of kindness and service helps both the person in need and me. I understand that it is only by God's grace that I stand in whatever shoe I have on today. This space and time allows me to flourish in a state of gratitude, which brightens every dark place in your life. Taking time to make these spiritual connections is like air and water. I take a deep breath and a long sip and stay connected through serving and giving.

Chapter 9

My family and friends are another huge component of how I care for myself. The truth is sometimes I don't know I need care. If it were not for being surrounded by people who know and love me, I don't know in what hole I may have ended up. Growing up, I watched my mother and her sisters come together every Friday at one of their homes. There was a pot of coffee on the stove and good casual conversation. They discussed everything from local politics and neighborhood rumors to what they were cooking on Sunday. But one thing that happened at 7:00 pm on the dot is one of the sisters picked up the phone and called "Mother." They spoke to their mother every Friday like clockwork. The phone was passed around to anyone who was in the house to greet and check-in on Mother. I never knew my mother and her siblings to allow any level of discord to come in and separate them from one another. This has been passed down generations in our family. Family connections and time to bond are extremely important to me. Moving away from the Midwest was very difficult for me because I missed all the impromptu family connection time, the holidays and birthday celebrations. It was so much a part of my DNA that once we had several other family members move to the area I adopted, plus a few friends, I started regular Sunday dinners known as The Gathering. Simply put, it is a way to stay connected physically, but more importantly, spiritually. Traveling with my family is something I love. I take a big trip with cousins every few years. This is precious time we spend creating memories, laughing, reminiscing, loving and exploring new adventures together.

My friends, the Final Few, as I lovingly refer to them, hold such a special place in my heart and in my soul. Truthfully, there's not room for many more who would fall into this category. Not the true, know all the details, lived it with you, friends. The Final Few are actually family. They know everything there is to know and, because of this, they are my safe place. That place where I don't have to be strong if I don't feel like it, but I know I'm protected. If you don't have at least 2-3 of these individuals in your life, you have some work to do. It's not a forced relationship, but a very natural state of being together.

Free my mind and my state of mind is a motto that I remind myself of regularly. Healthy mental and physical choices are essential for me. If there is anyone or anything getting in the way of my state of mind, I immediately work to remove it/them from the scene. Your headspace is just as important as your physical health. What I've learned from my 94 year old mother is don't stop moving, stay active, do something and that's exactly what I do. Spa time, yes, hair and nails, yes. If you don't feel good about yourself, do something about it. Where and how I spend my time relaxing is very personal. My husband likes walks in the park, I like walks in boutiques. It soothes me, takes my mind off the day-to-day, allows me to dream and shop from time to time. Being true to myself, and knowing what brings me joy and peace, is what I need. I don't explain or justify it to anyone else who is confused. It is my space, my time, my perfect peace.

Chapter 9

About the Author

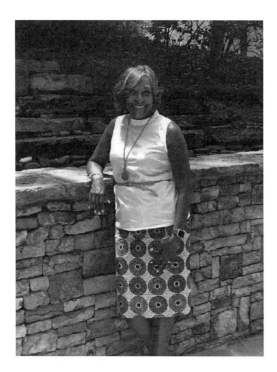

Turea Flowers, BS, SPHR is a native of Gary, Indiana and currently resides in Atlanta, Georgia with her husband of 18 years. She is the mother of three adult children. She has enjoyed an exciting career in Human Resources for more than 20 years. Turea began her career in retail, transitioned to the Financial Services industry and currently works for the fastest growing quick serve business in the United States. She is an active member of Women's Foodservice Forum, a 30 year member of Alpha Kappa Alpha Sorority, Inc., The PEARL Foundation and LinkedUP Church.

Turea enjoys time with her family, cooking, traveling and listening to live music in foreign places.

Contact The Author:

Email: tdflowers4u@gmail.com

LinkedIn: https://www.linkedin.com/in/tureaflowers/

CHAPTER 10

Let's Talk Rules

Where do I begin? I'd like to say that it all started when I was a little girl experiencing huge bouts of loneliness, or seeking to find a way to express myself; but I have always had a yearning for more within my soul. Sometimes people defer to it being from my obvious middle child tendencies, as I can, admittedly, fit quite seamlessly into the middle child stereotype. It's not hard when you have an older brother and a younger sister and grew up in a very Christian home. That's to say that this combination added to my desire to be an overachiever - at home, in church and, most definitely, in school. It also gave me an insatiable desire to have friends.

My, how I wanted people to like me! I was that little girl who would give up my own toy so that you would be my friend. Even as I write, I see the images repeating in my head - they're inescapable. "Give me your toy or I won't be your friend any more." Boom! Lightning speed, the other little girl could have my toy; she could have my vision, my destiny - whatever! Please, just take it and don't stop being my friend! Thirsty. I was parched, in a dry desert land wanting to have friends. While I think I've been able to manage to keep my head above water with this very real obstacle with which my life has presented me, I still think that there is an innate need inside of me - a desire to have people understand who I am. But living in New York City wrung that desire out of me.

More on that later. In hindsight, I think it's important for kids to have a tight family structure, and I did, though I remember plenty

Chapter 10

of times my friends were upset that I would choose a family dinner or a family outing over things like hanging out and drinking (this is a collegiate reference - when I was *almost* old enough to do so). In college, I was the "shiitake," as my mom says, because though we've let up on being super religious, cursing is still highly unacceptable in my household and I'd say that begins with the fact that my mom doesn't part her lips to speak a foul word. I used to curse with my Barbies when I was younger, so I heard it somewhere, likely from my Dad.

Back to college. It should be noted that I obeyed every statute - and there were plenty - that my parents established for me as the first daughter.

No boys.

No talking to boys on phones.

No boyfriends.

Therefore, no kissing.

No sex before marriage.

No hanging out with boys - they not tryna be your friend.

No sneaking out of the house.

NO.

Oh - no secular music.

Like a good Christian girl, I listened to every rule and then some. In fact, if I anticipated a boy wanting to do anything other than compare our pre-algebra scores, it would always be met with an absolute "no." When friends asked me about boyfriends, I'd simply say, "I'm not allowed to have a boyfriend." Call me brainwashed. But I think these policies worked out fine - for me. I know they're not for everybody, and my brother and sister didn't obey the majority of these rules outlined for them, similar to my own, especially the commandment deemed "no secular music." Yeah, that one wasn't about to happen. Bone Thugs 'N Harmony were at their prime during this time. I digress - again.

In obeying the rules, there was a bit of curiosity that percolated within me. Remember, I mentioned earlier that I always felt this need for more in my soul.

My senior year in high school, I had my first kiss - and it was on my 17th birthday after the Homecoming dance, which was my first dance I had a date. Cue the romantic Disney music, fireworks and slow motion. I was in heaven! After that, I had a slow incline in my guy game. My first boyfriend came a year later - and he was 3 years older - a 20 year old "man." Then came my college first "real" relationship that ended in sexual violation - that rule about waiting until marriage - absolutely broken. Then came several years of dating "men" that were no good for me or to themselves. Yet, somehow, the rules my parents established pertaining to faith - not religion so much anymore - kept me grounded.

One thing I want young women to know is whether your Barbies, imaginary friends, or real life friends and you curse, whether you're listening to Migos or whoever versus Mary Mary, you've got to start with you. That's to say, you need to know who you are. Where you come from. Have your spiritual rules. That way, you will not find yourself in relationships, whether romantic,

Chapter 10

platonic or familial, that result in you becoming a victim of being used. There are many ways to be used, and they start with how you use or treat yourself. After graduating with my Bachelor's in Theater at Santa Clara University in 2009, I moved on to work a total of four years before I decided to pursue my MFA in Acting in New York City.

The Big Apple.

To this day, I don't actually know what came over me - I guess I can say it is true that the older you become, the more afraid you become. This is often, in my opinion, mistaken for wisdom. However, in March of 2013, after years of being an unsuccessful people pleaser, performing in regional theater throughout the South Bay Area, and two years of working at Google - an inexplicable depression overcame me. It didn't exactly make sense, because I had the most ideal actor's life. I was working 9-5 at Google, performing in plays after work - sought after roles, too. First it was Beneatha in *A Raisin in the Sun*; next a Sharecropper in *Finian's Rainbow*. Then there was Treemonisha in *Tin Pan Alley Rag*, Maymie in *Intimate Apparel* and Nettie in *The Color Purple: The Musical*. Yet still, I felt quite empty inside.

It had been nearly one year since *The Color Purple* closed and there weren't any future shows in sight. I knew it was time to do something new. Later that day, I went to see *The Mountaintop*, which my friend and colleague directed. I went by myself and prior to the start of the show, Sam Cook's *A Change is Gonna Come* came on. I was moved to tears that I fought back with my entire being - I didn't want to cry BEFORE the play had even begun. As I flipped through the playbill, I saw "Master's." "Master's." Almost everywhere and it seemed next to everyone's name - the two cast members, crew - everyone seemed to have a Master's.

So, in that moment, I decided that I was going to pursue my MFA. After the play, I went home, told my family - and the next day at work, I applied to the only school that happened to still have open applications: The Actors Studio Drama School. At that time, one of my best friends was living in NYC and I had already purchased a plane ticket to visit her. I had also postponed the flight because of finances. Within two weeks, my reference letters were complete and I was ready to apply to school. I was invited to audition in May.

I arrived in NYC the evening prior to my audition. True story: I was so nervous that I couldn't memorize my monologue of a cathartic scene in *Ruined*. The next early evening during my audition, the words all of a sudden came to me. Every.

Last. One. My friend was my audition partner - that was how the auditions were structured. She was in awe of me – no, the God in me - recalling these words as they seemed to pour from a part of my soul that had not yet been touched. The audition was supposed to be approximately 15-20 minutes; it was an hour. They asked me to exit, I came back in and they offered me a seat in their cohort set to start in September 2013. It still gives me chills. I had been in New York for approximately 24 hours at that point, and I was already going to call it home. The beginning of my journey in NYC was full of butterflies, confusion, frustration, late night bar crawls with members of my cohort and JOY! I'm talking joy pouring from my heart, body, mind and spirit. Electrifying joy.

Chapter 10

Three months after the start of my first year, we were on holiday break and a mass email to my cohort got sent out presenting all actors with the opportunity to apply as playwrights in the program. If accepted, we would function as full time actors and playwrights in our three-year MFA program. A bit of back-story - the program at The Actors Studio Drama School is comprised of Actors, Directors and Playwrights.

One of the two playwrights in my cohort deferred and that resulted in them needing to fill at least one spot. I was selected as one of four actors to essentially "double major" (if you could) in Acting and Playwriting. I'd written throughout the majority of my life. Then, during a lull in my acting career, between 2012-2013, I established two blogs and a natural hair YouTube brand and channel. I was on fire. If moving to New York and going to grad school didn't slow down my pursuit of writing and producing, then my tasks as a master of acting and writing would be the ones to do so. Then life happened. Because, after all, I lived in NYC, and struggles in NYC wait for no one.

Less than 6 months after my move and these unforeseen opportunities, I met who would be my first NYC boyfriend, had roommate trouble, felt like my acting capabilities were always being overlooked and had forgotten about something that I've yet to mention to all of you - I was a storyteller.

The following year, 2014-2015, proved to be the most confusing and trying time since I moved to NYC. Wait - I think that is no longer true. Well...no. What doesn't kill you makes you stronger...errr...I suppose, so long as you don't take yourself out in the process. At the start of my second year in grad school, my playwright life began to really take precedence. Each second year student must participate in PDU, the Playwrights Director Unit. It's a class that is tucked away on Friday afternoons and lasts - what? Three hours? Yes, I believe it is three hours.

Wait. Let's take it back. In the spring of 2014, I conceived a play (that I have yet to give birth to in its full form - 4 years of artistic impregnation is rough) entitled *Sins Have Come: An American Story*. The exercise, or an entire year of PDU, is that each playwright collaborates with 1 - 2 directors to spend an entire SCHOOL YEAR developing a THIRTY MINUTE, ONE ACT PLAY. A moment of silence for the playwrights reading this that have their heads basically grazing the page right now.

You workshop this play EVERY FRIDAY, for the majority of a SCHOOL YEAR, to the same GROUP OF DIRECTORS AND PLAYWRIGHTS - and your instructor. Okay, for legal purposes, I'm going to go ON record and say any of the following - or the previous - is absolutely no shade to any parties or institutions involved in this process. This is my story...and you're still reading it, so enjoy the ride. Ah, yes. To continue...I workshopped this play every Friday, the majority of the school year, to the same group of directorsandplaywrightsandmyinstructor. Yes, that jumble of words is how it feels when you do this on repeat. The play suffered. I suffered. Then magic happened.

I suffered greatly. The play follows a biracial black man and his white half-sister in the aftermath of a crime. That's enough information - oh, the man is in denial of his battle with Dissociative Identity Disorder, previously simplified as "Multiple Personality Disorder" and in church as "he got demons." Truth.

Chapter 10

Kevin, the main character, and Jessica, the other main character, have only 30 minutes from beginning to end to go on a journey through my imagination, and that's a very interesting place to venture. Have you gone inside a middle child's imagination recently? No? Avoid it. So, for one year, they traveled through my imagination and as they got ripped apart - with love - and shred to pieces - with vigor, so did I, because I did not have the emotional maturity to separate them.

Oh, that boyfriend. He suffered. Or did I suffer him? Or did we suffer each other? Hard to tell when I was taking on the task of writing a play that led me to interview a criminal lawyer who practiced in Harlem, a nurse who specialized in mental health and reading endless scholarly sources straight from JSTOR. I was a mess. The play ended up being a success. Then, I was broken. Surrounding this chaos, I decided that I wanted to study Shakespeare at LAMDA - London Academy of Music and Dramatic Art - for one summer. I had never needed a passport; therefore, I had never gone to London. However, my same friend who lived in NYC and auditioned with me for grad school, now lived in London, 'cause she's a boss like that.

So, after 3 months of GoFundMe crowdfunding - I moved to London. Oh, well, for 5 weeks. I returned to NYC approximately one week before grad school was to resume - my final year. Why do I choose to relocate to places that are over 5 hours away within such a small amount of time? I don't like rollercoasters. So, perhaps, I love the rush of relocation. Regardless, I relocated, and then relocated again, and this time, I had a 4 week command of Shakespeare that New York could not offer me. Memories.

Lost 10 pounds simply because I drank real drinks and ate real food. And I was still - lost? Impossible. I know.

So, my third and final year of grad school began. I was wounded. Humans are mammals. That makes us animals. I'm a human. I was a wounded FREAKING (this is my Mom's book, so I dare not curse) animal! I'm telling you, 2014 - 2015 beat me up. I lost friends. I lost man-friends, or guy-friends trying to become men. I lost some weight. But I gained that all back by 2016. Lost my edges. Lost my esteem. Lost my vision. Then got a degree.

Oh, silly me. I also embarked on a very brand new adventure in my storytelling saga. I learned the art of SCREENWRITING. See, in our third year as playwrights at the Actors Studio Drama School, we studied screenwriting. That class saved me. No. Really - it did. I lived by myself from October 2014 - August 2017. I wanted my life to be - paused - by March 2015. Then LAMDA gave me something to look forward to.

Six months later, I began my last year of grad school - and that included screenwriting, which saved me. Perhaps it was the marriage of novel and performance. Or, it could have been something that had not yet been touched by human sins. But it was my outlet. My real outlet. It took off for me, I took off for it and here I am, more screenwriter than playwright, but proud of both forms just the same. I suppose we should fast forward to 2016 - the year of emancipation. I mean, the year I graduated grad school. Wait. This is accompanied with more struggle. Ah, heck! Let's get to it!

Chapter 10

In May 2016, I graduated with open wounds, scars that somehow couldn't QUITE heal, lots of knowledge, about 8 plays, one feature film and some short films - all in my back pocket. Still, your favorite middle child had no job. No job. A fancy Master of Fine Art - it sounds better if you round your few vowels there - but no acting reel. For you newbies, that simply means filmed - ideally, nicely filmed - proof that you can act. If you want to act on TV, you should have this, because people want proof that you can actually act on camera. Yhá Mourhia did not have this because she - I -- studied from a very theatrical performative history. Folks don't tend to record theater these days and, when they do, it tends to land in the archives at the Lincoln Center. A powerful, intriguing, accomplished woman who graduated in 2013 - the year I started grad school - encouraged me to just film something I wrote. That's a huge NO DUH moment. And I did. In September 2016, I filmed a screenplay adaptation of a short play I wrote entitled *Expulsion*. It was loosely based on my roommate history as experienced in 2014. We ran out of time and did not finish filming.

In November 2016, I began my production company, YháWright Productions! and launched a series called, *#LoveMyRoomie*, which was intended to be a short comedy based on the characters in *Expulsion* with pure intention to utilize the videos as fun back stories and encourage fans to donate - so that I could finish the film. In April 2017, I launched a crowd-funding campaign for #LoveMyRoomie Season 2, or #LMR2, and we didn't make any money. In May 2017, I scrapped the crowd funding campaign that I spent nearly 6 months planning and established my production company as Fiscally Sponsored under Fractured Atlas. Then folks donated 'cause their money was tax-deductible and I had more proof of concept. In other words, they started to believe I was serious. But we didn't make much money. In July 2017, I was tired of not being able to afford my rent, so I finally moved out of my apartment. In August 2017, I was homeless, with barely enough money to feed me until I got hired full time at a startup company in New York City.

In November 2017, I was promoted and received a healthy raise at my job. The date is July 24, 2017 as I write this. #LMR2 has received three festival Official Selection laurels - which means we're up for awards. I'm in pre-production for a short film. I'm in post-production for a short film I assistant directed and produced.

Next week, I'm on set for a new digital series, produced by Emmy nominated writers and producers. Y'all. My name is Yhá Mourhia (<-- that's all my first name) Dani'elle Wright. I'm from San José, CA. I'm a middle child and I talk to myself all day. Let's talk about the rules that you grew up with - yes the ones that sucked - and how you can use those rules to redefine your narrative and remove limitations. I urge every person who is looking for more focus in their life to hold onto some of my favorite rules:

No boys. I mean...they can be a huge distraction.

No talking to boys on phones. Long phone calls waste time when you could be working hard.

No boyfriends. If you have a significant other, make sure they support your dreams - like, for real. Therefore…

Chapter 10

No kissing. It's a gateway drug.

No sex before marriage. This might work if you're trying to stay focused on your dream.

No hanging out with boys. They not 'tryna be your friend - that's kinda true, actually.

No sneaking out of the house. Just take the key with you.

NO. Oh. No secular music - okay, Migos works.

I'm Gonna Let It Shine

She looks in the mirror, sticks her finger down her throat - you know where this is going. So, let me spare you the gruesome details but yes - I tried the majority of healthy and unhealthy weight loss plans. In high school, I cloaked myself in anorexia. I wanted to know what it felt like to starve my stomach down. Then I tried bulimia - the food I consumed was relentless and would not exit by human force. Of course, there were endless workout plans. Beach Body pilates, yoga, Tae Bo - all forms of Tae Bo. If you take it back even further than high school, in junior high, I was a B-Team athlete - a proud one at that.

I also survived off cheese bread, granola bars and an occasional veggie delight Subway sandwich because it was only about 400 calories, I believe. You see, we can go ahead and talk about burning candles, meditation, prayer, lip gloss made from bee's honey and bentonite clay masks because I've done that, too. But I want to be transparent with you - I'm talking, transparent AF. Self-care is not easy and yet it has become a buzzword in today's society. I'm happy to know that women of color are taking putting their glory on narratives that never existed and ensuring that the word becomes theirs. It's important for healing. We must remove these stigmas that plague our community and turn injured personalities into wounded souls. I've once almost been wounded. Yet, as with most of my life - the arts saved me. Now, I want you all to know that I'm not a natural hair fundamentalist. I'm simply speaking my truth, and you can disagree and turn the page, cut your eyes and continue to read, or hang out with me for a while longer.

Chapter 10

In 2006, during my first year of college, I decided to texturize my hair - yes, the Gerry curl. My understanding was that it helped your hair grow because of the moisture you had to maintain, and it was overall attractive because it took your naps and turned them into curls and waves. I'll never forget the day I cut my hair into a short haircut reminiscent of Halle Berry's. I wore a white blazer, white jeans, a pink and green floral shirt and green earrings and walked onto campus with this chic, short, curly cut. I mean, I was met with all sorts of positive reviews. Then I realized that though my hair was receiving positive feedback, my body - at a size 5 - was still too big. So, I continued to find ways to lose weight. Perhaps it was my youth, but the weight did fall off - the hair did grow but the esteem did not.

What does it mean to take care of yourself? Is it your nail color? Is it the cost of your pedicure or massage?

I'm here to say that I'm far from an expert, but after spending the majority of my childhood, and all of my adult years until 4 months ago, feeling like I was a prisoner of my body, I am here to say that self-care begins with the messages that you allow into your spirit, and more than anything, those that you tell yourself. My body is a temple. I was told this throughout my years in church and I've since strayed like a backslidden child and circled back to that which I know to be absolutely true. Your body is a temple. Your words are powerful. So, before picking up the book, signing up for the expensive classes and treating yourself to a mimosa, I want you to do me…no, you…the favor, and look inside at those desolate places.

Do you care for yourself? Because my experience is that in order for self-care to be sustained, it must start from within. This year, for the first time since my joy experienced on junior high B-teams, I've been the most consistent I have ever been with a workout routine. Not simply a diet - a workout routine. My place of work has provided me with the opportunity to join Orange Theory Fitness. You should certainly look into this place. It's intimidating and took me over ONE YEAR of contemplating to finally attend. This isn't sponsored content, so I don't want to speak on it beyond my jurisdiction, but I will say that this place has changed my relationship with my body. However, that's because through prayer and meditation, I began to change my relationship with my mind earlier this year.

So, what is self-care? It's those quiet moments when you might feel like you are going to scream. Be with that. It's those cookies when you have gone 6 days without any cheat meals. Perhaps, unless a licensed physician tells you otherwise, you should eat a cookie. It's massaging the knots out of your stomach instead of grabbing and shaking the fat. Shaming it. Shaming you. It's that walk to the park with your loved one. It's turning off Facebook notifications. Ignoring Instagram. Lying down on your bed and allowing yourself to just…cry. Then it's waking up in the morning and working out, challenging your body and sharpening your spirit. Self-care isn't yoga. But you can use yoga as a means to self-care. It isn't that hair appointment. But your afro looks good, sis, and that press has your hair swangin'.

For me, self-care is a journey, because as my life changes, my needs and demands for self-care change alongside it. However, what is always unchanged remains. I must love myself. Respect myself. Be honest with myself. Yes, even my darkness, so that I might see light. Commune with God when I need it most and when I don't feel I need it at all. When these and many other facets are aligned, I believe that we are all closer to the journey of self-care. It becomes easier to wake up and go to the gym. It becomes easier to turn down that bag of Cheetos.

Because you love yourself from within. Then, and only then, can your light shine so bright that you begin to even inspire yourself. This little light of mine. I'm gonna let it shine.

About the Author

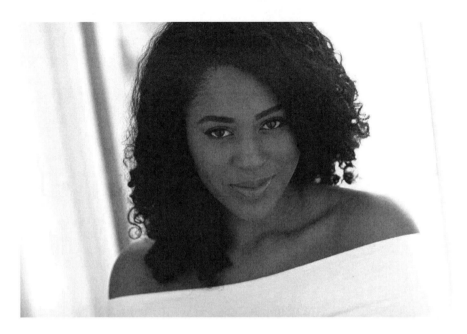

Yhá Mourhia Wright lives in Brooklyn, New York by way of San José, CA. After years of trying presumed setbacks and failures, she decided that she wanted to be an attorney. Much of her high school career was spent focusing on preparation for pursuing a law degree. It wasn't until her sophomore year at Santa Clara University that she realized her true passion was acting. It was during her sophomore year that she received a scholarship through the theater department. She was resolved in her passion and purpose and began onstage work in shows such as *Fuenteovejuna and Hair: The American Tribal Love Rock Musical*. In the years after graduating, Yhá Mourhia landed roles in renowned onstage shows such as *A Raisin in the Sun* and *The Color Purple: the Musical*. Soon maintaining wonderful momentum in Bay Area regional theater, she knew it was time to head for the Big Apple to pursue her master's and spread her wings!

Upon the start of her studies at The Actors Studio Drama School, where she pursued her MFA, Yhá Mourhia received the rare opportunity to study playwriting and screenwriting full time in addition to her acting studies.

In May 2016, she graduated with her MFA in Acting (whilst studying playwriting and screenwriting full time) and developed a diverse playwriting and screenwriting portfolio.

She is the creator/executive producer, writer and actress in her digital series ***#LoveMyRoomie***. In 2016, she established her production company, YháWright Productions! Her series, #LoveMyRoomie Season 2 (LMR2), has been well received by audiences and recently selected as an Official Selection in the Hip Hop Film Festival (Harlem), GLOW Television and Web Series Festival (Hollywood) and Newark International Film Festival (Newark, NJ).

Yhá Mourhia looks forward to the opportunities to continue her journey in storytelling, whether it is in front of, or behind, the camera.

Contact the Author

Yhá Mourhia D. Wright
Email: info@yhawrightproductions.com
IG: @mswrightontime
IG: @lovemyroomie
Website: http://www.yhawrightproductions.com/